95 - coffee
p.168 - for a list of
foods + pesticides

MW00897882

THIS BOOK CARRIES A 100% FEEL BETTER, LOOK BETTER AND LOSE WEIGHT GUARANTEE!

If you do everything in this book step by step and use the free resources on my website and do not feel better, look better, or still doubt the validity of this system, I will refund your full purchase price of the book. That's right. I will give you a full refund if this system does not work for you.

Ask anyone else with a book like this if they'll stand by their product like I stand by mine!

I want you to succeed and I know the information in this book will get you to where you want to go!

Visit http://www.LiveAwesome.com/book for all the details!

Hey Kevin!

I want to tell you that you've changed my life. Over the past couple of weeks I've really noticed how much my body, lifestyle and attitude has changed. I now exercise for at least an hour a day, 6 days a week and I really look forward to exercising. I get up and move as much as possible instead of sitting on my butt in front of the TV. I've also been eating REALLY well... Your Lifestyle Fitness and Goal Setting program really helped to put me on the right track and everything that's happened in my life since then has contributed to my success. I just want to thank you for your energy and motivation and to let you know that you've really made a difference in my life— something I'll never forget. :) You're great!!!

— Lisa, Golden's Bridge, NY

Kevin has helped me be more conscientious of what kind of foods I take in and portion sizes, too. I have begun taking different vitamins and have learned how to make yummy breakfast shakes! I was not normally a breakfast person, however I now take the time to make sure that I take part in one of the day's most important meals! The goal setting at first was difficult for me. I had to make this collage and stuff and I felt like I was back in elementary school! HA! I finally did it and did understand why it was important to have your goals made visual and put them out right in front of you...so you don't miss 'em!

I really felt that Kevin is one of the most dedicated individuals I know! I have learned a lot from his attitudes about health and fitness, but also about life in general. The funny thing is that even though I didn't work out with Annmarie once, I felt that I knew her well after a few chats on the phone and I always felt her energy and support! A great team!

— Melissa, Danbury CT

Annmarie, I do look good don't I! I'm so pleased with myself. I'm eating better and have more energy and I'm sure to keep exercising just for my health even after I've reached my goal which I'm not so sure what that is really, 145 was my goal at first but I'm not thinking weight so much now as I am fitness. But I'm happy knowing I don't need anyone to get me there but me, and of course a good trainer to show me the way to go. Thanks from my heart. See you on the 13th.

— Denise, Naugatuck, CT

Kevin, I just wanted to thank you for such a great program. It really fits my needs and my schedule. It's easy to do and I can do it at home or at the office.
Since we've last met, I'm back on a walking schedule and I've done your exercises. I've gotten back on track with my eating habits and started bringing a salad to work. I've definitely lost more than 2 pounds and am looking forward to losing more! Thanks again!

— Pat, Bridgewater, CT

Kevin and Annmarie,

You guys have not only helped me set fitness goals that I thought at one time to be impossible, but your kind motivation has moved me to start changing my negative thinking into a positive attitude! I now have clearly defined goals that I strive to achieve everyday. Your willingness to share your knowledge and experience has made it a comfortable and easy transition into a new and healthy lifestyle.

— Jaime, Bethel, CT

Until I went to the first Lifestyle Fitness Class, I was not happy, since I refused to believe after years of getting a Ph.D. in Shape, Self, People, Marie Claire fitness articles, I could possibly learn something new.

Fast forward an hour and a few sweat glands later: I was wrong. There was plenty I didn't know. But that wasn't because I was never told, I just never wanted to believe that I was doing anything wrong. This is how I'm made, I tell myself. I'm from a big family. I'm doing the best that I can.

These were all comfort zones for me, and that's where you guys came in: you challenged those comfort zones without alienating me, or turning me off from the program. Sometimes, we just need to talk ourselves out of our own complacency. It's good to hear other people working out their issues too, because even if it's not about the same thing, we all have those moments in our lives when we don't really know if we should, but know that we have to.

I walked into the class as a nonbeliever, but with each class, I was more and more convinced that if I kept up with the exercisers, managed what went into my body, and reminded myself of where I wanted to be, I would get there. Maybe not tomorrow, maybe not next month, but eventually, I will reach my destination. I know it's entirely up to me, and I have good moments and bad moments. And sometimes I don't want to do all 100 Hindu Squats. But now there is that little Jiminy Cricket (okay, so it's Kevin and Ann Marie...) saying, just a little bit, a little bit everyday, makes a big difference. And for once, I believe it.

Thanks so much for the class. I've taken more than you'll know out of it. I look at my collages every night (this time, no tears...) and I'm excited and thrilled that I've had the chance to spend a month focusing on what I want, physically and mentally. I look forward to taking the class in January that Ann Marie offers and hopefully by then, I'll be a little more flexible!

— Eileen, Danbury, CT

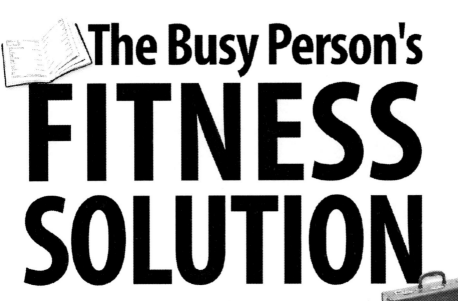

The Busy Person's
FITNESS
SOLUTION

THE OPTIMAL WELLNESS SYSTEM

THAT WILL GET YOU MOTIVATED, NEEDS A SPACE THE SIZE OF A BATHROOM

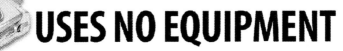

USES NO EQUIPMENT

and ONLY REQUIRES A FEW HOURS A WEEK!

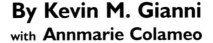

By Kevin M. Gianni
with Annmarie Colameo

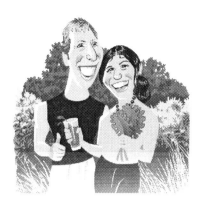

First Edition
Edited by Ron Martirano
Design by Thomas Morlock

A Better Life Press
P.O. Box 228
Bethel, CT 06801

ISBN: 978-0-9788123-0-0
Library of Congress Cataloguing Number: 2006908418

Publisher's Cataloging-in-Publication
      Gianni, Kevin M.
            The busy person's fitness solution / by Kevin M.Gianni ;
            with Annmarie Colameo. — 1st ed.
            p. cm.
         "The optimal health, fitness and motivational system
            that will get you awesome results with no equipment, a
            space the size of your bathroom and only a few hours of
            your precious time a week!"
            LCCN 2006908418
            ISBN-13: 978-0-9788123-0-0
            ISBN-10: 0-9788123-0-1

            1. Health. 2. Physical fitness.   1. Colameo, Annmarie.
            II. Title.

      RA776.G53 2006   613.7
                                  QBI06-600422

PRINTED IN THE USA

www.KevinGianni.com and www.LiveAwesome.com

MEDICAL WARNING AND DISCLAIMER

The exercises and advice contained in this book may be too strenuous or dangerous for some people, and the reader(s) should consult a physician before engaging in them.

If you experience pain while following this program, stop and consult a physician before starting again.

The authors of this book are not responsible in any manner whatsoever for any injury which may occur through reading and following the instructions herein.

Furthermore, the information in this book is not intended to replace a one-on-one relationship with a qualified health care professional and is not intended as medical advice.

It is intended as a sharing of knowledge and information from the research and experience of Kevin Gianni and Annmarie Colameo. We encourage you to make your own health care decisions based upon your research and in partnership with a qualified health care professional.

TABLE OF CONTENTS

Quick Fact:

Health Related Type 2 Diabetes Puts a $98,000,000,000 (Yes, Billion) Strain on Society and Our Health Industry... Yearly.

Statistic from www.obesityinamerica.org

STOP! Before You Read Any Further... Here Are Important Instructions on How to Use This Book

This book supplies the answers to great health and fitness in a way that you've never been shown before.

It challenges you to take matters into your OWN hands.

You're not 5, 10, 20, 30, 150 pounds overweight because of anything you've done consciously. No one wants to get fat. You've been confused and duped by misinformation that has made you fat.

Weight loss, fitness and great health are elusive, not because there's something wrong with you, but because of the misleading data and misconceptions that the food, fitness and health industry feeds to our hungry, "I've-gotta-lose-that-20-pounds-by-August" mouths.

So before, I unravel the lies and misconceptions you've been taught and unleash this new, revolutionary way to look at your own wellbeing, I'd like to give you these specific instructions on how to use this manual:

Instruction #1: Read This Book with an Open Mind

There are many things in this book that go against the information you're received in the past about health and fitness.

When I first started on my personal path to great health and fitness, I resisted the research I was finding and even my own experiences because the information was so different than what everyone had told me to be true. By doing so, it took me longer to get to where I am now—in great physical and mental health.

So if you want to get there right away, don't do what I did and resist.

Read the book with an open mind, use the systems I have put together for you, and start getting results immediately!

Instruction #2: Read a Chapter a Month or 20 Chapters Today

The intent of this book is to start you on a path to the great health and fitness you deserve. If you follow each step in the order presented, you will experience a dramatic change in your physical and mental being.

Though you don't have to go through the text systematically.

This book is also for busy people just like you, so I've designed each chapter to stand alone to give you the freedom to pick what you want without having to read the entire book. Each chapter will give you insight into what you need to do to start moving in the direction of optimal health.

If you want to jump into the exercising, go ahead. If you want to look at the nutrition information before anything else… it's there for you to benefit.

Just be careful. Each chapter will make you want to read more!

Instruction #3: Take Action at the End of Each Chapter

At the end of most chapters there will be a simple mental or physical activity that you can follow to solidify what you've just read. Once you begin to take action on these principles you will reach your goals. It's that simple.

There is a magic pill. But it's not 8-Second Abs or the South Beach Diet. The magic pill is ACTION. Take action toward your health and fitness goals everyday and you will get to where you want to go!

Don't waste your time reading if you're not going to do the follow-up activities.

Also, at the end of some chapters there will be a link to my information-packed health and fitness website. This regularly updated site is where the experts go to reveal their secrets on weight loss, longevity and optimal health.

When you type in the address, you will be taken to a special page that offers a free test drive of the site ($57 Value), where you can sign up and gain immediate access to the MP3 downloads, special reports, and videos.

You can also purchase an unabridged version of this book in audio format or download workouts and motivational programs.

There are two major reasons why this site exists:

1. Information always changes and I do not want this book to become outdated. With this site, I can constantly update my findings as new research becomes available, providing better product suggestions and overall recommendations to help you reach optimal health.
2. My goal is to reach busy people—and because I'm a busy person myself—I understand how the thought of a 700 page book can make a person cringe!

The website is http://www.LiveAwesome.com/book. I urge you to go there to find out more.

Instruction #4: Don't Listen to a Word I Say

What?!

Yes. Don't listen to a word I say. Once you've read this book take the information, use it and find out for yourself what specifically works for you and what doesn't.

I see and talk to many people who have opinions about things they know nothing about. This is their path. You can join them, or you can be a trailblazer and an evangelist for your own cause—your own health and fitness.

There are thousands of other books out there. This is just one of the many that will help you on your way.

Instruction #5: Smile

You're going to get to where you want to go!

QUICK FACT:

33% OF ALL CANCER DEATHS (185,757 OF OUR MOTHERS, BROTHERS, SISTERS, FATHERS, WIVES, HUSBANDS, FRIENDS AND CO-WORKERS ANNUALLY) ARE RELATED TO OBESITY, LACK OF EXERCISE AND POOR DIET.

Statistic from www.cancer.org and U.S. National Center for Health Statistics, Health, United States, 2004.

INTRODUCTION:

IT'S TIME FOR YOU TO TAKE COMPLETE CONTROL OF YOUR HEALTH... IF YOU DON'T THE STUDIES, GADGETS, MAGAZINES AND QUICK FIXES MIGHT END UP KILLING YOU.

Go to your bathroom mirror and take a long look at yourself.

What's happened to you?

You're heavier, you don't look as good as you used to and if you're like millions of others, you've tried with little success to get back to where you once were.

Wouldn't it be nice to hear that maybe the scientific studies, gadgets, magazines and quick fixes you've been given are all to blame for this? Wouldn't it be nice to hear that there is a mindset, some nutrition information and an easy exercise philosophy that actually works for busy people like you?

Well there is. And it starts right here.

It's time for you to take complete and absolute control of your own health and fitness.

This is why...

? **We've relied on scientific studies for the last half century to decipher what is healthy, what activities we should do and what should be on our dinner tables. Is it a coincidence that the number of fat Americans has grown exponentially over that same time?**

What has science done to you? What do you need to do to stop yourself from blowing up like a balloon on a helium tank?

You need to start taking your health into your own hands. You need to start going off on your own and experimenting with alternative solutions, regardless of what you've been told.

Within you lies the answer to vitality, energy and great health. You need to start exploring your options, outside of the contradictory scientific studies that tell you coffee is good for you one month and horrible for you the next.

Experiential knowledge is truth.

This book is an experiment. My partner Annmarie and I have gathered the information and techniques that have worked for us and the people we've touched over our combined ten years of experience in the fields of athletic rehabilitation, motivation and one-on-one personal training.

It is not exact science. It is undeniable, experiential fact that this is information that has made people happier, healthier and more vibrant.

In this book you will not be overwhelmed with scientific studies, as too often conflicting data is the result of bias. Figures and findings can be too easily manipulated to support pre-determined conclusions and funding sources, which is why I don't believe "flavor-of-the-month" reports will help you forge your own way.

One of the very few studies I'll mention comes from a JAMA (Journal of the American Medical Association) report, published in 2005, focused on the accuracy of medical studies. The results? You shouldn't rely solely on the findings of others to base your health decisions. Simply stated, travel at your own risk.

(You can read more about this study @ http://www.LiveAwesome.com/book)

What do you do now?

You start by reading a book like this that has you in mind. You're busy, you don't have the time and you run in 50 directions all at once.

This book is the first—and easiest—step to getting into great health and great shape. Why? It's going to help you find your passion for great health. This is the most important factor in finding your optimal health—having the drive to do so!

I want you to learn how to decide what works for you and I've given you the information that you need to get moving.

> **!** **I want you to stop listening to everyone tell you everything they know about eating right and exercising and I want you to start doing it your own way.**

What I want you to start doing is stop relying on the science and the articles that you read on CNN.com and the Food and Drug Administration (FDA) websites and start relying on the results.

Anyone can have a nice website, a few letters behind their name or a book with a nice cover. I have those things. So does the FDA. Do you believe me? Do you believe them?

It doesn't matter. You don't have to listen to a word I say. Nor do you have to listen to the FDA or the Center for Disease Control (CDC) or the American Cancer Society or the trainer at the local gym.

This book is cutting edge, front row information on how to live fit and healthy for this century and beyond. And it all starts with you—taking personal responsibility for your own health and wellbeing.

You can do what you please with the information here. All I ask is that you take action when you finish. Don't just read the book, put it back on your shelf and then do nothing.

Do something! Anything! I don't care if you throw a book burning party and toss each page into the bonfire. I just want you to take action.

You might find out some fantastic things about yourself that will change your health and fitness forever.

QUICK FACT:

98% OF ALL DIETERS GAIN BACK THE WEIGHT THEY'VE LOST.
90% GAIN BACK MORE.

Statistic from www.nih.gov

SECTION #1:

THE 7 BIGGEST HEALTH AND FITNESS LIES AND HOW THEY'RE KEEPING YOU FAT, UNHEALTHY, AND UNHAPPY

You've been lied to.

In fact, you've been lied to more than once.

Each one of these lies is stopping you from getting into the fantastic shape you've always wanted to achieve. There's a reason everything you've ever tried is not working.

The fitness and health information that you've gotten through the media channels—the magazines, the people you see on television, the reality TV shows, the gizmos, the gadgets—is old news.

It's stagnant. In fact, it's Flintstones-type technology that doesn't work in the real world. It's a complete fairy tale.

Why?

Because no one has taken a stand to say anything otherwise, no one's said anything that is so revolutionary and new to warrant enough attention.

The same old information in the books, CDs, DVDs, and workout programs keeps getting passed around like an old piece of Tupperware at holiday parties. It's the same information that's being taught in gyms, nutrition classes, courses and certification classes across America over and over again and it's becoming more and more antiquated as time goes by.

What is this information?

It's all the information you've ever heard. It's low-fat, high-fat, no-fat, high-carb, low-carb, some-carb-but-no-carb-what-the-heck-do-I-eat information. It's about drop-sets and dumbbell curls, egg whites and grilled chicken. You've heard it before. It's the information you've based all your past exercise and health programs on.

The certification text book I studied with to get my personal training certificate praised the food pyramid, preached the multiple benefits of the bench press, and was filled with guys from the '90's in muscle shirts and razor-cut Dennis Rodman hair.

The industry and government agencies are still passing this stuff off to you like it's the hottest and newest gadget in the store.

It's like a car dealer changing the sticker on a 1978 Chevy Nova and selling it as the 2006 model.

Or a real example… It took the FDA over 30 years to revise a food pyramid that everyone in the industry knew was making people fat!

How does being duped like that feel?

You think you have the newest, hottest, "this-time-I'm-really-going-to-get-it-right" information and it is just the same reworked, remodeled stuff that bodybuilders, trainers, nutritionists, dietitians and doctors have been using for years. And we're all getting fatter and fatter and fatter. It's a sham, and I'm here to expose it.

But before I give you the answers you are looking for, I have to admit, it gets worse.

Some of the people giving you the information KNOW that if you're duped and feeling confused that you're going to continue to look for more answers.

What does this translate to? Economically?

It means you're going to buy more products—more Ab-Rollers, more Gazelles, more exercise bands, more exercise balls, diet plans, books, more anything that they can sell as the new, next-best thing.

> **❗ The fitness and health industry is a billion dollar industry and it feeds off of your confusion.**

You've been there—I know, I have too. The same gadgets, books and DVD's are in my closets, too. These are all reminders of how we've been duped into thinking that if we just do this simple thing or use some easy system, we'll magically be granted all our health and fitness wishes. All in about 20 seconds or so, of course.

Let me ask you this…

> **❓ Would you go to a used car salesman to ask him for advice about how to get a good deal on a car that's sitting on HIS lot?**

No way!

So why do we listen to the magazines and the marketers?

They're one in the same. Without the money from the marketers who advertise in the publications, there are no health and fitness magazines. The more money the marketers make, the more they have to spend, and the more they spend, the more magazines there are to spit out old information and spin us in all different directions.

Yes, of course this happens in all industries, but the deeper issue underlying all of this is that people are getting hurt because of it. People are getting sicker and fatter because the information we're getting doesn't work.

This confusion must stop.

Depending on where you get your information from and who you talk to 50-75% of Americans are overweight. That's about 50-75% too many and it's my personal mission to change and de-mystify this industry, no matter what it takes.

> **!** **Every one of you deserves to know how to lose weight, how to feel fantastic and how to live vibrant lives.**

This isn't a low-fat plan, this isn't a low-carb plan, this isn't a Hollywood diet or 6-week transformation. This system shouldn't have any other classification except that it works for the people who use it—it's a lifelong wellness solution. You can call it what you want!

This is a system that opposes rigidness. It is meant for someone like you who is busy and wants to cut to the chase.

If you have some carbs, you have some carbs. If you eat some fat, you eat some fat. It's not a big deal. Fats and carbs both have essential places in your diet. There's no right or wrong with the information I give you. There is good, better, and optimal.

Each and every chapter in this book will give you an answer. There is absolutely no deception and no confusion. If you do everything I've outlined you will get the health and fitness you deserve. In fact, I guarantee it.

I will hold nothing back. And as I learn more, you will be able to visit my website *(http://www.LiveAwesome.com/book)* for the hundreds of pages of fresh and updated information that I couldn't possibly fit into this one book.

I'm here to give it to you straight. This book has the tools for you to succeed. You can build your health and fitness foundation one brick at a time or fill it all in at once and drastically change your life and your health.

To start, there is one thing that I want to make abundantly clear:

> **!** **You're not too busy for your fitness and health, they've only made it seem that way!**

You've been lied to and now it's time for you to take control of your own health!

Big Health and Fitness Lie #1: The Health and Fitness Magazines, Diet Books, Super-Bars, Protein Shakes, Gadgets and other Assorted Gizmos Are Here To Help You.

False.

These products are here to confuse you.

If you—and the millions of other consumers like you—figure out how easy it is to get into shape, the billions of dollars spent each year on gadgets, systems, trainers, and workout and diet plans becomes a trickle of pennies.

How many times have you wondered if the low carb diet is for you? How about the low fat diet? Do you know which one is better?

! **The heath and fitness marketers have made it so difficult to make any sense of what we should eat and how we should move that we're completely lost.**

It's not really in the interest of the fitness and diet product marketers—the ones that sell you books, magazines, products, and videos—to give you what you need to get into shape because then they'll have nothing to sell and nothing to promote.

Imagine if you were in the key and lock business and suddenly crime was eradicated. No one would need locks any more because their fear of burglary would be gone.

Same deal with the health and fitness marketers. If no one is afraid that they'll gain weight because they know all the right things to do to keep it off, those marketers are no better than the locksmith in the example above—out of a job.

Now let's put this into perspective. I'm talking about the marketers as a whole.

Does this make all health professionals bad, evil people? Absolutely NOT!

There are thousands of professionals out there fighting against the misinformation we've been fed.

But it does make you wonder how many people out there are playing with your needs when they promote their "New," "Radical," "Secret" or "Guaranteed" products, doesn't it?

BIG HEALTH AND FITNESS LIE #2: THE MODEL ON THE COVER OF VOGUE IS A PERFECT PICTURE OF HEALTH.

We cannot believe everything we see.

! **Models, fitness and beyond, are not the picture of perfect health. Supermodel Carol Alt—when she was in the prime of her modeling career lived on coffee and bagels. Arnold Schwarzenegger? Steroids.** *(Note: They were legal then…)*

What about the others? What about the guys you see on the fitness magazines? Do you really believe that they look like that under their clothes all the time?

They don't.

It is common knowledge in the training industry what some of these guys do to look like that for their photo shoots.

They bulk up and put on weight and muscle first by eating an exorbitant amount of food everyday—straining their digestive, circulatory, muscular and skeletal systems. Then they practically go on a starvation diet that gives them a minimal amount of nutrients. This is just a more intense version of binge and purge—over do it and then severely under do it.

Worse, in the last few days leading up to the shoot or body building competition, they drink barely any water (you might hold on to it) and stop eating anything with minerals that might cause the body to retain water.

And this is just if they do it naturally without steroids, HGH or any other muscle building, performance enhancing drugs.

Many of the fitness and diet programs you've done or read about are variations of this technique. You throw your body out of its natural balance for limited periods of time to achieve short term results through subtle deprivation or extreme overexertion. Is this what you want to put yourself through, only to briefly resemble a false ideal?

I know I don't.

You want fantastic health and fitness. The way of the cover model and centerfolds is all about smoke and mirrors. These images we're bombarded with are NOT real. The people are, but the message they are passing along to you is a lie.

Look at what's happening in our sports leagues. The players are getting caught using banned substances over and over again. Baseball is a mess, so is sprinting, and so is cycling. What other sports are passing along this lie?

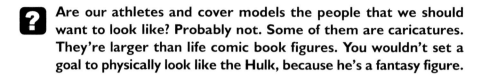

Are our athletes and cover models the people that we should want to look like? Probably not. Some of them are caricatures. They're larger than life comic book figures. You wouldn't set a goal to physically look like the Hulk, because he's a fantasy figure.

Just as fantastic are the images we see everyday on our TV's, magazines, and the internet. Don't buy into this and you'll be happier, healthier, and more successful than you'll ever imagine!

BIG HEALTH AND FITNESS LIE #3: SCIENTIFIC RESEARCH SHOWS...

Buy into the back and forth of the "flavor-of-the-month" scientific studies and you'll crash and burn.

I've done it. So have you.

If you really want to rely on science, You have to look at who's doing the study, who's funding the study, how many people participated in the study, how controlled the study was, and if they did a follow up study to verify results.

This is a daunting task and if you actually take the time to do so, you'll find that many of the studies are much more inconclusive than the media reports.

! **There is one scientific fact about exercise and health that you need to know. The fact is this: if you start to take control of your own health and fitness you WILL succeed.**

You might think that's not exactly science, but it really is. I remember reading Newton's laws in the 7th grade: "For every action there is an equal and opposite reaction." Translated to fitness: For every action you take there will be a reaction that will give you feedback and tell you if it works or if it doesn't.

You can't listen to all the studies that say working out at a certain time of day is better than another, or doing this type of exercise is the ONLY way to get the results you want. There is no "only" way. There are ineffective ways, there are better ways, and for each individual there may be a best way.

For an "only" to exist, it must be an "absolute," and if an "absolute" keeps changing, it's absolutely wrong!

You don't need doctors and physiologists and trainers telling you what is right and what is wrong, or what has been scientifically proven and what hasn't.

There's a 10,000 year history of exercise that we've completely ignored over the past 30 or so years that has all the answers you'll ever need.

The lessons from all these years are based on common sense. Move, move and, yes, move—and do so sensibly. It's so simple it pains me to tell you.

Note: In this book, I will teach you some metabolic science because it has worked for me and my clients and many of the trainers and mentors I've learned from. It works because it is complementary to our natural biological processes.

The system is Fat Burning Heart Rate training. It is simple and you can use it with any activity you do, without a heart rate monitor or any fancy equipment.

Is it the absolute answer for everyone? No, but if you try it—you will lose some weight and feel fantastic.

BIG HEALTH AND FITNESS LIE #4: YOU MUST WORK OUT 7 DAYS A WEEK FOR 30 MINUTES EACH DAY...

...If you're a robot.

I laugh when people say you should exercise six to seven days a week for at least 30 minutes. Not because it's bad advice—it's just not realistic to start.

When I hear this, I get a silly image of cavemen logging their 30 minute cardio workouts on their cave walls.

They just didn't do it. They just moved. That's all they did and it's all you have to do too, in terms of exercise.

So if it's not six to seven days a week for 30 minutes, then how much exercise is the minimum you should be doing?

Three to six hours a week—anytime. Just move when you feel like it, rest when you don't. It's that simple. This program will give you all you need to know about how, when and where.

And if you're good at math and saying "wait a minute, those numbers are just about the same," then you're right. They are. But it's all about perspective. This whole book is about changing your perspective.

> **!** **If I tell you that you need to workout for seven days a week and you miss two days, what happens? You realize you've created an impossible goal.**

Eventually you'll lose some steam and start to feel bad that you're not sticking to the program.

Further along in this book, I've laid out a simple way for you to keep track of your activity using a point system instead of hours. All you need to do is accumulate a certain number of points a week and you're on the fast track for fitness success. You can use it or you can keep track of hours, just don't get caught in the "number of days" exercise trap.

When you keep track of points instead of days you never set yourself up for failure. If Friday rolls around and you have 30 Points to accumulate, your goal is still possible. You can squeeze in 5 points after dinner or 25 points on Saturday morning....

You won't believe how easy it really is.

Big Health and Fitness Lie #5: No Pain, No Gain

I thought this saying went out with the bodybuilding craze of the 80's, but I am still amazed to hear people mutter those 4 words in the middle of a tiring workout.

You know you shouldn't be hurting, you know that the "no pain, no gain" philosophy is wrong, but you're still pushing too hard.

 Pain means stop.

And this is exactly what I make sure anyone I'm working with does when they're in pain. I want you to do the same.

Your body diagnoses what's going on inside with extreme efficiency. If something smells, you don't eat it. If something tastes bad, you spit it out. If something rubs, you get a blister.

If something is getting damaged, you feel pain.

Why on earth do we continue to push through this pain?

There are probably a few reasons. One that I think is most revealing is that we've applied a mental ideal or construct to combat a physical fact.

If you're a salesman and you don't like cold calling, but go out and call 1000 people, you'll most likely be rewarded by more sales, a bigger paycheck and a nice new car. That makes sense. This is the mental "No pain, no gain." You have to break out of your comfort zone.

But on the physical side, pain is a fact—not a mental construct. If you have pain in your lower back, there is actually a physical issue, muscular or skeletal, that needs attention. If you keep doing whatever it is that is hurting you, you will eventually do irreparable damage.

The salesman isn't in this type of danger—he just doesn't like making phone calls. This is an emotional belief or a discomfort, not a physical fact. He will not tear a muscle and not be able to physically walk away from his desk if he makes a couple of calls.

 An important distinction between pushing mentally and pushing physically is that your body has limits, your mind does not.

If it hurts, don't do it. Assess if you're doing it right, and then try it again. If it hurts twice, give it a rest and maybe try again another day.

Don't force your fitness and risk an injury that could damage your body and interfere with your health and fitness for the rest of your life.

BIG HEALTH AND FITNESS LIE #6: RUNNING AND WALKING ARE HARD ON YOUR KNEES.

Revised: Running and walking incorrectly in poorly designed shoes are hard on your knees.

If we weren't supposed to walk and run, we wouldn't have legs and feet. Our bodies don't have wheels. We have legs and feet and toes and they all play an important part in our locomotion (the way we move).

Put those feet and toes into a pair of poorly designed shoes and suddenly the foot gets dumb. Worse, over time, we get bunions, our toes overlap, and our arches collapse. Each structural failure builds on the next, destroying our natural shock absorbers—our feet—and changes the way we walk.

I want you to find a shoe right now and take a close look at it. Compare it to your foot. Looks different, right?

? **Why on earth do we need a shoe with a padded rubber heel that is over twice the width of our own human heel? Are our heels not good enough? Is our design inherently flawed?**

The shoe companies have made you think that this technology transcends nature—that it is a necessity to have padded feet with monstrous heels. What they haven't told us is that it's causing us to walk incorrectly. Those heels are hurting our knees, hips and lower backs.

! **Millions of people are in pain because there's no one to tell them that they've been feed a marketing message that is fallacious. What's worse is that our doctors and physicians have been sold on it as well.**

They're the professionals telling you not to run. Not to walk. Not to do one of the most efficient, fat-burning activity of them all. No wonder you're confused. These are the people we've been told to trust.

But don't blame them. They're not at fault, and they're definitely not out to hurt you.

Doctors and physicians are specialists in their particular fields of medicine. They have been trained to treat and diagnose illness. Some have been trained in preventative medicine and fitness that they pass along to their patients.

Does that mean they're running and walking experts? Not unless it's printed on their diploma (or other certifications). If they're not working in their area of specialty, then chances are they haven't done much testing and training with people to experientially know what can be accomplished by even the most debilitated people. So they pass along the misinformation they've heard from magazines and studies and we do what they say because—as a society—we generally believe what our doctors tell us to do.

What I'm saying is not a knock on the medical field, it is an observation. I'll be the first to tell you that you still need to trust your doctor, but at the same time start taking control of your own health and question what you've been told.

BIG HEALTH AND FITNESS LIE #7: SET REASONABLE GOALS BASED ON YOUR LIFESTYLE IN ORDER TO SUCCEED.

Translation: Set the benchmark low, because there are more important things in your life than your health.

! **No wonder we're fat. We've put our health on the backburner. If you don't think that your health is the absolute most important thing there is, you better rethink your goals.**

Yes, goals do work. In fact, a good portion of this book is on goal setting, visualization, looking at your past success and making your goals a reality.

But when I hear that in order to succeed you have to shoot for the moon, when you could have the stars, I cringe.

Do you think star quarterbacks set goals to win 5 or 6 games in a 16 game regular season?

Do you think CEO's tell the board that they're planning on being just a little bit in the red?

? **Do you ever get in the car and head out to the grocery store, then turn around because you're satisfied you've made it halfway?**

Then why is everyone in the health and fitness industry telling you that you should compromise your own optimal wellbeing?

! **Your health and fitness should be the most important priority in your life. Without it, you cannot do ANYTHING, because you're DEAD.**

NEVER compromise your health goals. As far as I know, we only have one chance here on this planet, so don't listen to someone who thinks you should live a mediocre and half-baked life.

I want you to make your goals big and take big action. Don't be reasonable.

It's your life, live it with excitement, great health, fitness and vibrancy!

QUICK FACT:

SALES OF PACKAGED SNACK FOODS IN THE US TOPPED $61,000,000,000 (BILLION) IN 2005.

Statistic from www.marketresearch.com

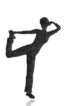

Section #2

The 8-Step Process That Will Prepare You to Soar Beyond the Health and Fitness Goals You've Been Told You Could Never Achieve

> *We don't exercise our million-dollar body because we have to work fifteen hours a day at our $60,000 a year job.*
> – Jon Gordon "The Energy Addict"

Before I get into the details of this 8-step process, I need to address something very important—your priorities.

In order for this, or any, program to work, you MUST be willing to make your health your FIRST priority. Why? Because, to use a title of a book by the nutritionist, Jane Pentz,

? "If you don't take care of your body, where are you going to live?"

I believe this to the N-th degree...

All the worrying you may do—about making money, being a good parent, having fun, getting a raise, achieving your ultimate goals—means NOTHING if you are neglecting the vehicle (your body) that allows you to do all those things.

If you are unhealthy, chances are you are less likely to balance your life to achieve all your goals, less likely to be a wonderful, caring and responsive parent, and less likely to have money, business and personal success you desire.

People who neglect themselves by not eating properly, not exercising frequently, and not following through on their health and fitness commitments are people who will not see the maximum potential of their own energy, vitality, and success.

Your life accomplishments are directly linked to your abilities to manage your own health and fitness.

Since you need to make your health a number one priority, let's look at it from the perspective of another habit you've grown accustomed to over the years. Showering.

 I've always been fascinated with how we Americans will go to tremendous lengths to clean our outsides when our insides are as nasty as the local dump!

Most Americans shower daily. When we were children, we were told that you must keep yourself clean in order to fight off disease and, of course, be able to talk to other people without offending them with your stench. Even the dirtiest of people manage to shower once in a while, right?! Why? Because they are aware of the necessity to keep themselves clean.

People always find the time to shower. It's already built into their day. They do it in the morning, or in the evening. Some women (and men as well) can take not only an hour to shower, but an additional 1-2 hours getting their hair ready or putting on make-up. I'm sure this hits home to some degree, whether this is a friend or it happens to be you.

In terms of cleanliness, showering is good for the exterior of your body. And as Americans we have this down to a science. We have body lotions, deodorant soaps, shampoos, shampoo-conditioners, conditioning shampoos, hair gels, body perfumes, etc. Chances are you have one or two—if not all of these products in your bathroom. I know we do! But again this is cleanliness on the OUTSIDE.

In terms of cleanliness for the INTERIOR, our best option is a well-balanced mix of mental growth, exercise, eating habits and detoxification.

Now here's the disconnect between showering habits (outer cleaning) and exercising/healthy habits (inner cleaning). Depending on where you get your information, you'll find that at least 25-40% of all Americans are sedentary. Sedentary means that a person has NO leisure time activity. Not once a week, not once a month. Sedentary means NONE. This would be the equivalent to never cleaning the INSIDE of your body, EVER!

What does this mean? It means that 25-40% of Americans are FILTHY ON THEIR INSIDES! And those who only exercise once or twice a week are pretty dirty as well, even if they eat relatively decent foods. Why even bother showering, when your insides are neglected every single day.

Your insides are much more important than your outsides.

Your cells, organs, muscles and bones have no chance of survival if you do not keep them healthy by exercise, diet and self-improvement. Cleaning yourself externally by showering and facial creams will only remove some bacteria, oils and sweat.

Cleaning yourself internally will actually give you more benefits in terms of appearance than a bar of soap and moisturizing cream. People who are hydrated properly and eat many water containing foods like raw vegetables and fruits have healthy, shiny skin—the same type of skin that a topical can only hope to emulate!

 For some reason or another, someone dropped the ball when it comes to informing us that we need to take care of our bodies and that cleanliness starts from the inside. Anything else is just the same as the cover up women put on their faces—a quick fix.

Put the ball in your court and become aware of your body and how it reacts to exercise and the food you eat and you'll notice a huge difference in how clear your skin looks, how toned your muscles start to become, and how much energy you seem to still have at the end of the day! This is something worth working out for!

» ACTIVITY » "GET YOUR PRIORITIES STRAIGHT!"

Take a few minutes to think about your priorities. List your 3 most important priorities below and give a reason why they are important to you. Are they kids? Family? Job? Money? If health and fitness is not one of them, then I'd like you to think about why it isn't, and how you can make it one.

If your physical and mental well being is not one of the top three, you are not giving your priorities their greatest and best attention. By not taking care of your health and fitness, you are not functioning at your maximum level of energy to give your other priorities their fair share!

Priority: _____

Reason this is important to me:

_____

_____

_____

Priority: _____

Reason this is important to me:

_____

_____

_____

Priority: _____

Reason this is important to me:

_____

_____

_____

MIND WORKOUT STEP #1: HOW ONE OF THE WORLD'S MOST WELL-KNOWN TRAINERS PREPARES HIMSELF FOR ANY SUCCESS

» ACTION » SMILE.

 What would you attempt to do if you knew you would not fail?

— *Robert Schuller*

The simplest thing you can do to start achieving your goals and being successful in your fitness and health is to stand up straight and smile.

That's right. It is that simple.

Your physiology is how you represent your physical body to the outside world. Smiling not only tells people that you are happy it also sends signals to your brain to produce endorphins that physically and mentally make you feel better.

Along with this happiness and better mood comes confidence and assertion. When you are smiling you can make better decisions and accomplish more.

Tony Robbins, probably the most well-known motivational speaker in the world, believes putting yourself in a good mood, with a gesture as simple as a smile, can gear you up for fantastic success.

Think about all the great businessmen and woman and politicians that you've seen on TV and, if you're lucky, in person. Most of them all have very powerful presences, right?

When I was younger I met Joe Lieberman, the Connecticut senator and 2004 Vice-Presidential Candidate. Even though he is very short and some people might say not so attractive, he radiated this very powerful energy that was definitely a projection of his inner "state." He was smiling, standing up straight and very confident.

Your state is what makes your emotions. If you are smiling and breathing deeply and fully you are most likely in a good state. If you are frowning and slouched in your chair, you are most likely not in a productive or pleasant mood, or bad state.

ЭЭЭ

> *When people come to me and say they can't do something, I say 'Act as if you could do it.' They usually reply, 'Well, I don't know how.' So I say, 'Act as if you did know how. Stand the way you would be standing if you did know how to do it. Breathe the way you'd be breathing if you did know how to do it right now.' As soon as they stand that way, breathe that way, and put their physiology in that state, they instantly feel they can do it.* —Anthony Robbins, Unlimited Power

Tony Robbins writes in his book Unlimited Power, "When your physiology runs down, the positive energy of your state runs down. When your physiology brightens and intensifies, your state does the same thing." When you make an effort to change your physiology, you can instantly change your emotional state!

» ACTIVITY » THE SIMPLE 15 SECOND, 8-STEP EXERCISE YOU CAN DO ANYWHERE THAT WILL MAKE YOU BEAM LIKE A KID ON CHRISTMAS... ANYTIME OF THE YEAR!

(Yes, put the book on the table where you can read it, stand up and do this exercise right now!)

Follow along step by step for this to work...

1. I want you to stand up from wherever you are sitting now. When you stand up, don't stand up straight. I want you to slouch.
2. And when you're slouching, I want you to put a frown on your face.
3. While you are doing this for a couple of seconds, I want you to try to think about something that is really happy.
4. Pretty difficult, right?
5. Now I want you to stand up straight.
6. Put a smile on your face. I mean a really, really big smile!
7. Now try to think about something that is sad or upsetting.
8. It's almost impossible! I know every time I do it, I can't even begin to think about something sad... and even if I do think about something sad, I don't see it as that sad when I'm smiling.

This really is too easy!

Think about how this can change your life! If you start changing your physiology now and use that tool when things get rough, you'll be able to breeze through hard times with a smile and great posture!

When you are in line at the post office and the counter person is chatting with a customer for what seems like hours and you're in a big rush... smile, breathe deeply and fully and stand up straight. Notice how different you feel. It doesn't bug you as much.

Apply this to your fitness and health goals and you're already off to a fantastic start! When you don't want to exercise because you're sitting on the couch and watching TV... sit up, smile and breathe naturally. I guarantee you'll begin to feel like getting up and moving around.

When I write, I have to be careful, because if I get into too much of a happy state, I have to get up every 5 minutes because I have so much energy!

Let me tell you just how powerful this is. If you've heard of Norman

Cousins (Anatomy of an Illness), then you know the true value of changing your physiology. Cousins made a remarkable recovery from an illness by using laughter. He would spend a good deal of his day watching funny movies and reading funny books that immediately changed his state. Once his state was changed, remarkably, his body used his new energy to heal itself!

Keep this in mind while you are reading the rest of this book. If you are sitting up straight and smiling, then you will be setting yourself up for a fantastic experience. If you are not, then you are compromising your fitness results.

For more simple tricks to put yourself in the best mood ever, visit http://www.LiveAwesome.com/book.

PHENOMENAL HEALTH AND FITNESS SECRET
SEE YOURSELF FIT, HEALTHY, AND HAPPY, AND YOU'RE JUST A STEP AWAY

Some people think this secret is voodoo.

They say, "you can't imagine something and then have it just happen."

I'm here to tell you that this is one of the most carefully guarded secrets in all industries. If you can picture it, you can become it. There are thousands of books on this, and each and every one of them tells the story a little differently.

The one glaring similarity is that when you follow the instructions of these books and manuals and visualize your goals, things will happen that you never thought were possible.

I hesitate to explain this further, because I'm not sure how it works. It defies logic. We're taught in school and beyond that hard work gets you to where you want to go. It does, but sometimes hard work isn't enough. I know people who push themselves in the gym and try to focus on their eating, but they still can't put it all together and lose the weight.

When I get those people as clients, I realize that they really can't believe and see themselves at the weight they want to be. It's only a number on a scale to them—not a picture, not a feeling.

You have to be able to see, feel—and almost touch—yourself as a slimmer, healthier and happier person to ever get there.

MIND WORKOUT STEP #2: WHY THE TOP FITNESS AND HEALTH PROFESSIONALS ARE IN GREAT PHYSICAL AND MENTAL HEALTH AND YOU'RE NOT.

» ACTION » LEARN TO VISUALIZE YOUR SUCCESS

Unless you try to do something beyond what you have already mastered, you will never grow. — *Ronald E. Osborn*

You've seen them in the magazines, in the tabloids, on the covers of their own books.

They're all in great shape and you've listened to what they've written, but you still don't look like them.

Why is this? They know something that you don't know and they're not spilling the beans.

 Trainers and the top fitness professionals are in great shape not because they're going to the gym seven days a week (although many do) and it's not because they're eating right (although they are). The reason they're in great shape is because they've visualized themselves in healthy and fantastic shape. Once they did that, the rest fell into place.

Maxwell Maltz wasn't a fitness professional at all. He spent most of his career as a plastic surgeon changing the way people looked. He found that many of his patients did not need plastic surgery... **they just needed to change their image of themselves.**

So instead of always putting his patients on the operating table, he started to work with changing their self-image. Many of the patients he worked with began to realize that they really didn't need to have surgery. They just needed to change the way they viewed themselves.

His work is called Psycho-Cybernetics. It was published in the 1960's, but is still very prevalent today. Why? Because it works!

To apply Maltz's ideas to fitness are simple… you have to see yourself in shape and accomplishing your fitness goals to be a success. Visualization is the key to making your goals come to life.

You should spend time thinking and visualizing yourself as healthy, fit and energetic.

Picture yourself smiling and taking a walk, or picture yourself with a six-pack of abs. Once you make a habit of this, your self-image will shift from how you view yourself now to a new self-image that takes on whatever traits that you envision.

Regardless of your objective, for the best results you should visualize the steps it will take you to get there. Imagine yourself moving along your path and picture yourself at different points along the way. Picture yourself losing 10 pounds, then the next step may be losing another 5. The clearer the picture, the better your chances of reaching your goal.

If you'd like to be skinny and in shape with defined muscles, think about how you will act, how you will talk to people, what you will say and how you will feel. You eventually will start to do the things that you've visualized and know you are on the right track.

» ACTIVITY » THE TWO MINUTE, LOOK-LIKE-A-FITNESS-PRO VISUALIZATION EXERCISE

Take a minute or two tonight before you go to bed to think about how you want to feel once you start focusing on your health and fitness. Imagine how you'll walk and how you'll communicate with other people. Try to imagine yourself doing things that someone who is in great shape would do. Spend a little bit of time there. If you like what you see, and we know you will, then do this a couple nights a week. You can do it everyday if you like. Make it a habit and you will succeed! I promise!

MIND WORKOUT STEP #3: EMBRACE FAILURE AND LOSE WEIGHT QUICKER THAN YOU EVER THOUGHT WAS POSSIBLE

» ACTION » LEARN TO FAIL

One mistake doesn't mean failure, and one thousand failures do not make for a lost cause.

Edison did thousands of experiments when he was trying to invent the light bulb. With each one, he came closer to his goal, by learning what did and did not work in his efforts to make the bulb stay lit!

Ever been on an airplane? Well what would happen if you got on a plane with no destination? That would probably be a bad idea. Eventually that plane would run out of fuel and you'd better hope there's a really big field below.

Same deal with visualization. If you don't have a clear picture of where you're going then you're going nowhere. If your plane is going to Miami from New York, the pilots will navigate it southward and eventually get it on course with the runway for landing. Is it always going in the exact direction of the Miami airport? No. It is constantly adjusting to get there.

Your path to success toward a goal is like the plane's route home, requiring constant readjustments until you're safe on the ground. If you find yourself off course, stopping the journey before you get to where you're going isn't an option.

! **View diversions as readjustments and you will reach your goals quicker and happier.**

Here's a great story a coach of mine, Nick, once told me about failure and success.

There was a young boy named Michael, about ten years old, that Nick had been counseling for a short period of time. Michael was overweight and was having a difficult time at school. He had trouble with his math and was a level or two behind in reading. He just didn't feel good about himself and the other kids were starting to pick on him because of his reading deficiencies and, of course, his weight.

Nick had met with Michael a few times and now the issue they were discussing was his performance at school. After pulling some teeth to get Michael to talk about his problems in school and with the other kids, Nick was unsure of how to proceed with the session. So he asked Michael a very blunt and straightforward question. "How do you feel about yourself?"

Michael responded with this, "I feel like a big fat failure."

"Whoa, hold on a second," Nick said, "What makes you feel like that?"

"I don't know, I just am."

Nick, knowing this wasn't going where he wanted it to go, smartly changed the subject quickly.

"Well Michael, tell me about something that you really like."

Michael looked up to the ceiling. "I like animals!"

"And tell me, what's your favorite animal?"

"The Cheetah!" Michael nearly jumped out of his seat.

"Great!" Nick matched his enthusiasm, "and tell me about the cheetah."

In double-time, Michael began to tell Nick all about the cheetah, how it walks, how it eats, how it sleeps, when it sleeps, again what it eats—to the point where a non-caring Nick would have kicked himself for asking this question at all.

When Michael seemed to be winding down, Nick gently interrupted.

"Wow, you certainly know a lot about the cheetah don't you? You mentioned something that I want to talk about. You said that the cheetah eats zebras, right?"

"Yeah, and antelope, and..."

"Well, Michael, when the cheetah goes out and hunts, how many times does he get the prey so can eat dinner?"

Michael thought for a minute then exclaimed, "All the time!"

Nick's face became more serious, knowing Michael was wrong and he slowly gave Michael his lesson, "That's not true, Michael. The cheetah is lucky if he gets to eat once or twice a week. He hunts many times and doesn't catch a thing. Did you know that?"

"No, I didn't"

"Michael, the cheetah is a very special animal because it keeps trying all the time, day after day so it can eat. He may miss his dinner four or five times in a week. Now would you call the cheetah a big fat failure for not being successful every time?"

Michael got the lesson and started performing better in school.

We can't be at our prime all the time, and when we aren't, we absolutely cannot punish ourselves for it. Be more like the cheetah—go out everyday knowing that you are doing what you need to be successful.

Let's face it. You cannot do everything perfectly.

So while you're following our program, I want to give you one permission above all other permissions. I want to give you the permission to screw it up. I want you to make a mistake. I want you to "fail" a few times.

And when you do, take a minute, hour, or day, to breathe, look over your goals and then refocus your concentration. For many of us, fitness and health require a lifestyle change that creates LASTING habits! You're bound to slip up once in a while, so don't be hard on yourself.

 Learn to fail and learn that failure is another way to learn.

» ACTIVITY » HOW TO BE A CHEETAH

Here are the tools that will allow you to be the Cheetah you've always wanted to be!

Step One: When you start to think you're failing at something, listen to what you're saying to yourself. It will probably be similar to things like this, "You stupid..." or "I don't believe you just..." or "Why can't you ever keep a commitment for..." For this step, just listen and be aware that this is happening so you can recognize it when it happens again.

Step Two: Tell yourself that you are thankful you are having these feelings. Seriously. Even if they're very self-degrading. Thank yourself for sharing your thoughts because regardless of how nasty you are to yourself, you still have to appreciate everything... the good and the negative.

Step Three: Take a few deep breaths.

Step Four: Ask your conscience to move on to the next thought. Some people say "Cancel," others say "Thank you for sharing." Whatever you like will work! If the next thought is just as negative and just as degrading, repeat the four steps!

When you master this, you will be able to deal with your negative thoughts and "failures" easily and quickly before you begin to start the self-doubt that can destroy your chances of reaching your ultimate fitness goals!

MIND WORKOUT STEP #4: STOP YOUR THOUGHTS FROM MAKING YOU FAT

>> ACTION >> COOPERATE WITH YOURSELF

>> *'Getting it together' requires slowing the mind. Quieting the mind means less thinking, calculating, judging, worrying, fearing, hoping, trying, regretting, controlling, jittering or distracting.*
>> – W. Timothy Gallwey

Your head is stopping you from getting into great shape. I guarantee it.

! **The only way to accomplish your goals is to learn how to cooperate with YOURSELF!**

One client I had used to stare blankly between sets of exercises. It was a deep and intense stare into space, and after seeing this happen during our first few sessions together, I asked him what he was thinking about during his tune-outs. He told me he was thinking about work, something that I later learned he always thought about.

Do you think he had the most focused and effective workout when his mind was somewhere else? Not a chance.

W. Timothy Gallwey wrote a fascinating book in the 70's about how to play "yoga tennis." (The Inner Game of Tennis) No, this is not a creative way to use the "Downward Dog" position to strengthen your serve and volley game, it is a way to view the game and the inner chatter a player experiences on the court while he battles an opponent—or in Gallwey's view— themselves. Though Gallwey moves through different aspects of the game of tennis like strokes, form and how to win, his words beg to be interpreted into everyday living.

Gallwey speaks of two "minds", the conscious self (Self 1) and the unconscious self (Self 2). Self 1 always tends to be hard on Self 2. "You are doing it all wrong," the conscious Self 1 might say. Or "Your push-up form looks worse than your grandmother's!"

Can you think of a time when you've had this type of self-talk?

I think many more of us encounter this EVERY DAY!

Ask yourself this:

 Is your mind-chatter making you second-guess your success?

The trick to conquering your mind and reaching your goals is to let the two selves function in harmony, which requires you to stay present at all times during your workouts and hopefully beyond!

So stop thinking and start doing!

The quote at the beginning of this chapter talks about how to get it all together in your head. It's all about letting Self 1 and Self 2 working together. I've broken each aspect down so you can start getting them together and get your fitness goals in line!

Stop judging yourself against others and yourself.

When you are exercising or meditating or doing anything, do the activity with little concern about how you are doing it or if you are doing it correctly.

When you practice less judgment you will find you are not so hard on yourself anymore and that you can reach your goals quicker. Ultimately, you will have more finishes than unsuccessful tries. If you do find yourself judging, address Self 1 and Self 2 and say: "Let's be gentle on ourselves and work together toward our common goals."

Stop allowing the inner chatter.

When you are exercising, make sure that you are only doing the exercises. If you find your thoughts wandering to the future and about a meeting you have after lunch or that the cats need to be fed, gently bring your thoughts back to where you are.

This is a peaceful practice. Tell yourself, "Come back to now." When you learn to control your thoughts, you will find you have much more peace and quiet. You will certainly have less stress, because you will deal with things in the present when you are supposed to deal with them—NOT when you are exercising!

Stop figuring things out, calculating, or trying to think in the future.

If you calculate, you are not thinking in the moment. You are thinking slightly in the present. Since we are speaking of tennis in this chapter, I can tell you that I've had many potential great shots hit the bottom of the net because I've calculated where they were going to go, before my opponent's ball even hit the court on my side.

When you stop calculating, you will be in the present and you will focus more on what you are doing instead of strategizing. In terms of your work-outs, you will need to stop planning ahead—stop thinking about how many reps you have left and how long you will wait to do the next set. This is strategizing and calculating.

A part of me would almost prefer you to not even count reps, because it will stop you from thinking about finishing and interfering with your actions. The other side of me is very aware that counting the number of reps is a great measure of success and progress. Considering this, I'd say that the benefits of self-monitoring outweigh the liability. So for now still keep track until I can find a better way!

Stop worrying... about EVERYTHING!

When you are worrying, your mind is very far away from the present. If you are worrying about your progress through this program, tell yourself that you are doing wonderfully, you are doing great things and you are on your way to accomplishing all you've set out to do. If you doubt yourself, you will struggle and this will be miserable. I am sure that if you were doing this to be miserable, you would have found some workout program that promises unattainable goals and 5-second workouts. You are doing this to do some-thing remarkable for your life and the people around you. Smile, relax and stop worrying. You've already made it this far!

Fear and worry are similar. Generally what you worry about is the fear of something. You need to stop letting fear get in your way of your successes. The more you fear failure, the less you will accomplish in terms of your fitness. When you find yourself in a difficult time and you know you are fearful, tell yourself this gently: "I will not let fear control my decisions. I will succeed!"

Stop hoping and trying. Start doing.

The words "hope" and "try" are non-committal words. When you hope, you are not doing anything, you are just thinking about being positive. There is a difference between "thinking about being positive" and being positive. If you hope that you will lose weight, you are not taking any definitive action, you are just thinking about taking a definitive action. Instead of hoping, actively make a difference by taking action. Don't hope to lose weight, tell yourself you will lose weight and then take an action that supports losing weight. Make a commitment to the action and you will put yourself in the best position to see it through.

To "try" is the same thing. Trying is a non-commitment to an action. When you say that you'll "try to workout tomorrow," you are setting yourself up to miss working out tomorrow. When you don't make a solid commitment, your mind and body act accordingly. They will take minimal action to make you a success.

Great athletes and people who are in shape do not hope or try. Many of them have eliminated these words from their vocabulary. Imagine Michael Jordan, in an interview before the NBA Finals, saying, "Well, Bob, I hope we can win this series. I know I'm going to try to make some baskets and try to help the team win four out of seven." No! He's going to say, "We're ready for whatever they throw at us. This is the goal we set at the beginning of the season. We're prepared to give our all and we are prepared to win!"

So when you think of trying to do something, think of Michael Jordan or any other professional athlete saying that he or she is trying or hoping that they will succeed. You'll probably give yourself a good laugh and get back to accomplishing your fitness goals!

Stop regretting.

Regret is a sign that your mind is in the past, not the present. You are aware of only what has been. If you are regretting past workout failures, you are setting the blueprint for just another unsuccessful attempt. If you are regretting that you missed a workout the other day, you are bringing your energy down just enough to miss another one because you are feeling bad about yourself. People who succeed and are fit and have wonderful health, do not regret the mistakes they've made. They build on them and come back stronger.

Stop controlling.

When you try to control your success you are setting yourself up for disaster. (Notice the use of "trying" here.)

Most "Diets" are people trying to control their eating habits. When you are dieting all you do is cut down on what you eat and temporarily control your urges, which is why you are generally unsuccessful. Did you ever notice that there are some people that are always on diets? You may even be one of them. Those who succeed when they diet have done more than control their food intake, they've created enough action and motion towards a goal that they do whatever it takes to lose the weight. They make the commitment that this is for the long run and that they've set a goal to complete it and it means something.

You can never accomplish something solely through control. Athletes do not control the outcome of a game, they do their best and if their teammates are doing the same, generally the team wins!

Less Distraction

Each of these examples serves to distract you from your goals. If you can work on eliminating the behaviors that interfere with your fitness successes, then you will be healthy, have more energy, and be able to set new goals that you are confident you will be able to accomplish!

For even more advice on how to take care of these pesky thoughts, visit http://www.LiveAwesome.com/book and get a free copy of the "Excuse Busters" report!

» ACTIVITY » TAKE COMPLETE CONTROL OF YOUR MIND CHALLENGE

I want you to be aware of the times when your mind is trying to sabotage your success. When you catch yourself being fearful, being distracted, or worrying, I want you to be gentle and say to yourself this general affirmation: "I appreciate that (these) thought(s), and now let's focus on what happening right now."

(When you use the above, or if you decide to make up on your own affirmation, be sure to always thank yourself for your negative thoughts before you bring yourself back to the now. It is important that Self I knows it is appreciated in order for the two selves to work together!)

I want you to take a day to be aware of your inner chatter. Bring a pad around with you if you like and take note about what you were thinking about and when. Then come back to this workbook and fill in the sentences on the next page by writing down four our five times when you caught yourself out of the now, not just when you were working out, but anytime. Write what you were doing, when you caught yourself, what you told yourself to stop the thoughts and if the thoughts were suppressed.

The First Time:

Today I caught myself _____

when I was _____

When I caught myself, I told myself to _____

_____

and afterwards I felt _____

The Second Time:

Today I caught myself _____

when I was _____

When I caught myself, I told myself to _____

_____

and afterwards I felt _____

The Third Time (Wow, I Never Knew I Did All These Things!):

Today I caught myself _____

when I was _____

When I caught myself, I told myself to _____

_____

and afterwards I felt _____

The Fourth Time (I Really Do This a Lot!):

Today I caught myself _____

when I was _____

When I caught myself, I told myself to _____

_____

and afterwards I felt _____

MIND WORKOUT STEP #5: YOU'VE BEEN THERE BEFORE, WHAT MAKES YOU THINK YOU'LL FAIL NOW?

» ACTION » THINK ABOUT AND WRITE DOWN YOUR PAST SUCCESSES.

If you take too long in deciding what to do with your life, you'll find you've done it. — George B. Shaw

---

The only way you've achieved any success you've had in your life is by making commitments.

When you make a commitment to anyone, including yourself, you have now made your goal and it can start happening.

I'm sure you, just like everyone else, have your share of successes to date—maybe you've gotten a degree, started your own business, just got a raise, or wrote a book. I don't want to hear anyone saying they can't think of anything!

Many different people have varied views on what is successful and what is not—for some success is raising a wonderful child or making a 15-layer chocolate cake, for others it is completing a 20-story apartment building or flying around the world in a hot air balloon!

❗ It's not important how others view your successes, what's important is how YOU view them. Anything you've committed to and completed is a success!

I was working with a client who needed to lose a substantial amount of weight--about 80 pounds. She was a young and motivated business owner who started her own private practice in her mid-twenties—a real strong young woman.

Her challenge was that she was afraid of starting to lose the weight because she thought she was going to fail. Sound familiar? Just about everyone can understand this at some level. So I had her list her past successes in her workbook.

Surprisingly (not to me, but to her), since high school she's been a success at EVERYTHING she's done. There wasn't a year unaccounted for that she wasn't successful in something that she started.

I pointed this pattern out and she recognized it. Then I asked her, "You've been a success since high school, what makes you think that you're going to fail now? You haven't failed at anything in eight years!"

She understood.

? **Too many times, we can base our emotions and feelings on unfounded principles. What have you thought that you couldn't do before, but then realized you were just making your own road blocks?**

Your past success can be the framework for your future success. Why? Because with each past success you've had, there have been ups and downs, times you wished you could quit and times you felt great.

When you look at what you've done before, you can use your past accomplishments as reference points for what you are doing now.

Here's an example:

My college graduation was a big deal for me. I label it as one of my more significant successes. In those four years, there were times I wanted to quit, there were times when I had a blast, and then there were times when I questioned what I was doing in school in the first place.

Each one of those things I felt along the way toward graduation was all part of the larger picture or goal, which was the college diploma I received when I reached my goal.

You see, every path to reaching a goal is different because different things, emotions, and circumstances factor into your achievement.

Though, when you look at it more closely, every path towards reaching a goal is SIMILAR because of the similar feelings that arise. Let me explain.

On the path to reaching any goal, everyone feels doubt, excitement, fear, questioning. It is natural. So when you think about reaching your goals you have to build in the structure--or know that these things will happen and that you can overcome them easily.

That's why looking at your own past successes is so important. By taking a past framework or structure of a goal that you achieved you can actually see the times that you wavered and when you waiver while you are attempting this new and present goal, you will not get too discouraged because it is part of the process.

I apply my past success in college to many things. When I set a goal to run a race and two months before the race, I don't feel like continuing with my training, I'll just think about the time I finished college and that there were plenty of times that I didn't want to go to class anymore.

Eventually I got back on track in college, and with that knowledge in hand, I know that eventually I'll get back on track with my training schedule and run the race that I set my sights on.

The middle of every successful project looks like a disaster.
— Rosabeth Moss Cantor

To see my own rap sheet of failures and successes, visit
http://www.LiveAwesome.com/book and have a laugh on me!

» ACTIVITY » START GETTING THE RESULTS YOU DESIRE TODAY WITH "MY PERSONAL PAST SUCCESSES WORKSHEET"

So speaking about successes, I'd like you to take a few moments here to brainstorm and come up with at least seven successes that you are proud to write down on paper. If you think seven is a bunch, think harder, they are there... you just haven't thought of them as successes.

Did you live up to a promise you made to someone? Did you keep a really private secret for someone who trusted you with that candid information? Did you reach a goal in business or your personal life?

With each of these seven, I want you to then give a reason why you view this as a success.

Here's an Example from my own Personal Success Worksheet:

Success #1: Graduation from Marist College

I'm Proud of This Success Because: I managed to accomplish this milestone through some of the hardest, most exciting times of my life. I remained committed to this degree for four years even though there were times when I wanted to outright quit and go off and do my own thing. This success has given me job and career opportunities that otherwise would not have been available to me. It has also given me the strength to push through other commitments I've made and make them successes as well.

See how it works? Good, let's turn to the next page and get started. Be sure to really get down to the heart of why you think these are successes and write more than just a sentence or two. You will call on these later if you hit a bump in the road in your fitness and health training. Take as much time as you can with this exercise. The more time you really think about what you are setting out to do, the better the results!

Success #1: _____

I'm Proud of This Success Because: _____

_____

_____

Success #2: _____

I'm Proud of This Success Because: _____

_____

_____

Success #3: _____

I'm Proud of This Success Because: _____

_____

_____

Success #4: _____

I'm Proud of This Success Because: _____

_____

_____

Success #5: _____

I'm Proud of This Success Because: _____

_____

_____

Success #6: _____

I'm Proud of This Success Because: _____

_____

_____

Success #7: _____

I'm Proud of This Success Because: _____

_____

_____

The exercise you have just completed is the first exercise in this step. On the website, I have posted an exercise that will straighten you up and get your mind more focused than it's ever been in only 20 minutes. Plus it will help you lose weight while you're doing it! Visit http://www.LiveAwesome.com/book to get a move on it today!

Mind Workout Step #6: The Simple Reason Why Over 97% of People Fail... You Might Be A Victim of it Already...

» Action » Find Out What You Really What to Accomplish

 Unless you try to do something beyond what you have already mastered, you will never grow. — *Ronald E. Osborn*

Find out what you REALLY want to do and you will succeed.

Have you heard about the Yale Class Study of 1953? An entire class of Yale students was asked if they had sat down and actually set goals for their future. Only 3% responded that, yes, they did. Only 3% of *Yale* grads! When they were revisited many years later... that 3% of students made more than 50% of the total money made by the ENTIRE CLASS!

So be a Yale student that sets goals when it comes to your health... imagine how much energy you'll have! If the numbers are the same, that means you'll have 50% more energy than all of the other people in this world combined! Well, maybe 25%. I say this half kidding and half very seriously!

 The reason people are adverse to setting goals is because they associate them with failure.

They have set themselves up for failure before they have even started out. Not that they intended to do this, but because they didn't know how to put together a strong set of goals that are attainable and motivating.

Now let me let you in on a secret that is going to change your goal setting for your entire life:

 You need to set goals that really get you pumped if you ever want to succeed!

I have this set of CD's from T. Harv Eker. I don't even know what the title of the program is, all I know is that when I'm sick of talk radio (which usually takes around five minutes) I pop one in and listen to what he has to say.

So I'm listening to Harv in the car and he says something that I have to repeat. So I scan the CD to find it again. When I repeat it, I get the chills...

He says, "everything you've ever done in your life has brought you to the point you are at right now."

Let me say that again... "everything that you've ever done in your life has brought you to the point you are at right now."

Make sense? Maybe it's not so ground breaking for you, but I want to explain what it meant to me and I think you'll take something from it.

I spent most of my life in fear of how people would react to anything I'd say. I was afraid of the word "no." I was deathly afraid of rejection of any kind.

Some of you might be able to relate. That fear lead me to a place where I had no self-confidence, no money and where I was always feeling trapped. Every decision that I had made that avoided the possibility of hearing "no" lead me straight to an unhappy, miserable place.

It was torturous. I was there for a while.

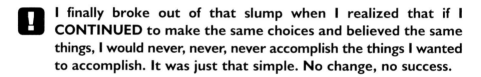

I finally broke out of that slump when I realized that if I CONTINUED to make the same choices and believed the same things, I would never, never, never accomplish the things I wanted to accomplish. It was just that simple. No change, no success.

This applies to you in thousands of ways. If you are overweight, tired, worn out, angry, anxious, in a dead end job, in a dysfunctional relationship, etc., then your decisions and beliefs have brought you to that exact place. Similarly, if you are broke, lazy, fearful, your actions and thoughts have brought you to that exact place.

You've created this reality for yourself. Like Eker says, everything that you've ever done in your life has led you to the point you are at right now.

When you see it this way, it gets you thinking.

Here's the kicker: if you continue to believe the same things and take the same actions, you will continue to live the same overweight, tired, worn out, angry, anxious, in a dead end job, in a dysfunctional relationship, etc. life that you are living now.

There is no magic pill.

If you rate the quality of your life on a 1 to 10 scale (10 meaning fantastic) and it is not a 10, then you have some serious decisions to make. I don't know many people who are striving to live a "5" life, but I'll bet many of you have that rating for one or two aspects in your life. If you don't start to change the way you think and act, then your "5" will ALWAYS be a "5".

Since you're here for health and fitness, let's think about it this way... if you are out of shape and can't find the time to exercise even though you really want to... that's fine... just know that your decision is based on your present beliefs, not new ones that can propel you into a life of energy and vibrancy.

If you are addicted to sweets and you know that it brings you down, but you always make up the excuse that it's just how you are, then yes, you will always be the same—addicted to sweets, worn down and gaining more pounds.

You need to start breaking free of your past beliefs.

I spent years breaking free of the negative belief systems that were installed in my head when I was younger. I would always look at the negative, before I looked at the positive. ALWAYS. When someone would present an idea, I'd say "What if _____ won't work because..." etc. The negative ruled and it got me nowhere!

Maybe you're like this. Maybe you have different challenges that you need to think about. Anger, anxiety, fears, health, relationships...

! **Start questioning your belief systems by doing things that are out of your comfort zone. Start by doing the opposite of what you normally would do. Start by smiling and taking fear with you... not letting it stop you.**

You should be living a "10" life, full of vibrancy, energy and creativity. You deserve it. Start shaking it up today.

If you set a goal that does not juice you to a level of 8 or more, on a scale of 1-10, I'll tell you right now you've already failed.

You know why? Because you don't really want it! Anything that is not an 8 (even 8 is pushing it) or higher isn't important enough to you. You might as well find something else that is a 10 for you to focus on. But when you do, let me tell you this, if your health isn't taken care of, you aren't giving what really juices your undivided energy. Why? Because you get more energy from fitness and health to do the things you really want to do!

» ACTIVITY » WHY THE HECK ARE YOU HERE AND WHAT DO YOU WANT TO ACCOMPLISH?

So let's see how juiced you are about your health, so we can weed out those of you who might be unsure that you want to live with your life energy soaring and feeling better than a million bucks!

When you set goals make sure you examine yourself and your reasoning. Go deeper than a superficial "I want to lose weight." Here's why:

Lisa was working with me over the phone and we had just finished most of the program, when she told me that she still wasn't finding the motivation to exercise. I asked her what she thought the issue was and she told me that she gets too distracted during the day. She's a mother of two and has to do everything that a stay at home mother has to do—drop off and pick up the kids, clean the house, pay the bills, do the dishes, etc.

Her goals of losing 10 pounds and feeling better just weren't motivating enough.

So after a few phone conversations and a little more frustration on her part, I told her that there's got to be something more important than losing the weight. Just like a flood gate, she opened up and told me just how important her children were to her and how important it was for her to be a fantastic example for them. When she didn't have any energy or wasn't smiling it wasn't fair to them.

So we adjusted her goals to focus on being a fantastic parent. Guess what… she lost the weight in no time, her husband had never seen her smiling so much and her kids were excited to have their energetic mommy back!

Are you ready to set the goals that are going carry you far beyond what you've accomplished before? Goals that are going to give you energy for life? I think you are, let's take this on with energy and excitement.

I want you to look back at the "Start Getting the Results You Desire Today with 'My Personal Past Successes Worksheet'" and pick 2 or 3 that you are super-proud of. These you will write below. (What?! You didn't do that exercise? If not, just think of three past successes that you're proud of! Your fitness depends on it!)

Successes that Make Me SUPER-Proud!

1. _____

2. _____

3. _____

Now I want you to think about the steps you took to accomplish these goals. This will help you realize that each success is a series of tiny motions forward.

Your exercise and your fitness are just like this, tiny steps forward to living a fulfilled life with bounds of energy. What's nice about this exercise is that you can think about a success and then apply it to your fitness. I like to do this with my fitness and apply it back to my career and other things.

For example, getting back into running shape after an injury I once had was difficult. There were many days I wanted to stop running because I was winded or whipped. If I had stopped, I would not be here telling you about it.

Each time I kept going, I created a base for the next day that I ran, which was just a little bit easier. Then the time after that was easier still... and so on.

So why don't you breakdown one or two of these successes so you can see all the steps it took to get there.

Steps That It Took For Me to Achieve Success:

_____

_____

_____

_____

_____

_____

Great! Now let's set your goals for your fitness and health!

» ACTIVITY » BRAINSTORM, PRIORITIZE AND ACTIVATE YOUR MAXIMUM POTENTIAL

Before we go any further, we need to figure out what you want to do! First you are going to write a list of 20 items that you want to achieve from your new level of fitness and health. Examples could be: More energy, stop drinking coffee, feel better in the morning, lose 10 pounds, have rock-solid abs, cleanse my body, etc. This is a brainstorming session, so let it fly. If you get stuck, keep pushing for more... I'm sure you'll get them all out.

1. _____
2. _____
3. _____
4. _____
5. _____
6. _____
7. _____
8. _____
9. _____
10. _____
11. _____
12. _____
13. _____
14. _____
15. _____
16. _____
17. _____
18. _____
19. _____
20. _____

OK, now you have a really long list of things that you want to accomplish with your health.

I wouldn't be surprised if you've done this before. Most goal setting starts like this.

The sad part is that this is also where it ends—as brainstormed ideas on paper. Nothing tangible, nothing that really will move you to accomplish what you set out to do. This list of twenty things you've just compiled is destined to fail if you leave them like this. I guarantee it.

So now it's time to get excited about making goals that will last and leave a lasting impression on your choices for your entire life! I want you to go through these items and rate each one in terms of your motivation to accomplish them on a scale of 1-10 ("1" meaning you could give a darn, "10" meaning this is really what I want to do). You can have as many 10's or as many ones or anything in between, just be honest and don't think about your ratings. Just mark them right next to the line it is on.

Here's an example. My list includes "run longer distances." I'm psyched to push my body to its limits and accept that challenge for my self at any time. So I'm going to mark this one with a 10. Get it?! Go ahead and mark 'em up!

PHENOMENAL HEALTH AND FITNESS SECRET

MAKE A HABIT OF SMALL DAILY ACTIONS AND YOU'LL NEVER FAIL WITH YOUR HEALTH AND FITNESS

Do something.

Do something small everyday and you'll suddenly have big results.

It doesn't matter what it is and when you do it. If you move once, twice, six times in a day and do it everyday you will lose weight and feel fantastic.

You need to make a habit of action in order to reach your goals. Take action today and see results tomorrow.

I'm a runner. When it's time to run, I get my shoes, my water, my running belt, car keys and walk out the door. I don't think. I do.

When people ask me how I can run 40-50-60 miles a week, I tell them that it's easy. I just go. I stopped thinking about it a long time ago.

You should start doing the same thing—instead of thinking about exercising and how you should do it, just start moving.

Do it now. Find a bookmark, get up for 30 seconds and march in place.

It feels good doesn't it? Now string a couple more minutes of that together and take a walk after dinner and you're off to a fantastic start.

This book will give you options on how to move, so you won't need to guess what you should do and don't end up just swinging your arms around in a circle or wiggling your toes (though that is a start!).

You can of course go beyond my suggestions as well—all I want you to do is start moving and the rest will follow.

It's supposed to be simple. Don't resist this advice!

Mind Workout Step #7: Learn the Art of Laser-Like Focus

» Action » Find Your True Motivation

 If you have the will to win, you have achieved half your success; if you don't, you have achieved half your failure.
— David Ambrose

Everyone has some type of goal right? If you've done the exercises I gave you in the last activity, you might even have twenty. So how do you start achieving them?

You need to make them invincible.

Making your goals <u>Invincible</u> requires three things:

First: You need to weed out the ones that are just flak.

It is silly to try to focus on too many things when it comes to fitness and health because your energy can be compromised.

You wouldn't want to try to become a better long distance runner at the same time you wanted to be a power lifter as well as a semiprofessional basketball player. Each one of these activities takes up a bunch of time and it's pretty much a given that sooner or later you will get burned out! So pick two or three that are best for you.

Many goals are complimentary to each other, making them easier to group together. Loosing weight and running a 5K are great together. Learning gymnastics and increasing your flexibility are actually a MUST to have together!

So when you weed out your goals, try to maintain complimentary objectives and take massive action. Your focus will be clear and you will accomplish what you set out to do. You will have plenty of time to tackle the other ones once you've breezed through the first round.

Second: You need to make them specific by assigning a who, what, where, when.

If you are not specific, you will not reach your goal.

I will say that again.

If you are not specific, you will not get what you ask for.

Why not? Because if you have no idea where you are headed no one else does either.

If you say you want to lose weight that's great... until you only lose one pound over two months. When what you really wanted to do was lose 25 pounds over four months!

Making goals specific is the who, what, where and when. What exactly is your goal, who is involved in your goal, where will you be accomplishing your goal, and when do you think you will accomplish it?

Using one of my personal goals, I'll illustrate what I'm talking about.

One of my "10" goals is to "run longer distances." Well that's great, but how much longer? And by when? So let me be more specific. "I want to run a 50-mile race by November, be prepared to do so and do it with ease and healthy joints."

I've now set myself up to do these things.

If I focus on just running a 50-mile race, then I might do it in 20 years. If I focus on just doing it by November, I might not be prepared and I might hurt myself. When I include those specific instructions, then I will be almost guaranteed that this will not happen.

When you make your goals specific, you are helped along with intention, just as long as there are specific instructions.

Third: You need to bring them home by answering the question "why?"

"Bringing your Goals Home" means that you have to put an emotional attachment on them.

You now have to think about why you really want to achieve that particular goal. Why is this goal important to you? Why do you want to accomplish it? Why do you want to have more energy? Why do you want to lose weight? Have more time? Eat better?

This is where Lisa's story from a few pages back really comes to light. Why did she want to lose the weight? When you've identified this simple reason, you're on the path of least resistance!

 You will struggle achieving your goals if you don't ask yourself why you're striving to reach your health and fitness goals.

This step will give you the strength to continue when you hit rough spots. It will keep you motivated for extended periods of time.

Let me show you how to do this with my goal. I had "run longer distances" then got more specific by changing it to "I want to run a 50-mile race by November, be prepared to do so and do it with ease and healthy joints."

Now I ask myself why.

My reason is because: "I love the challenge of pushing myself and I get a wonderful feeling when I am running outside in nature that reminds me of how remarkable life is." Sound convincing?

Maybe you think it's crazy, but guess what I'm thinking about every time I go out for a run? I'm thinking about how wonderful it will feel when I'm running though the canopy of a trail, breathing in the fresh air and stopping for a sip of water just around mile 35. Your goals may be similar to this one, they may be much different.

Say your goal is that you "want more energy" and you've made this a 10. Now to be specific, you need to say that you "want more energy so you can spend more time with your three year old, or you can stay up later at night and read without feeling too run down to do anything." That's pretty specific.

The next step is to ask yourself why you want to spend more time with your three year old. For you it might mean that you can share the joy of having a wonderful child who lights your life when he smiles. This is bringing it home. Whatever reason moves you will allow you to accomplish any goal you set. This is where you become invincible.

 You will not be stopped if your reasons for success are close enough to home to make you feel something inside!

>> ACTIVITY >> WEEDING OUT YOUR GOALS FOR MAXIMUM FITNESS SUCCESS

In the previous Activity "Brainstorm, Prioritize and Activate Your Maximum Potential," you made a list of goals and assigned them numbers on a 1-10 scale. What really juiced you was assigned an 8 or higher. Now let's look at those goals again and decide which ones you want to achieve first.

All of these goals that have high rankings are fantastic to have and what you need to do is pick the most important to you so you don't have too many things to focus on at once. By focusing on only two or three goals your attention will not be spread too thin.

To weed out your goals from the previous exercise, I want you to take your list and copy everything rated 8 or higher here. I imagine you have about 3-5. If you have more, then only take the five highest. If you have less, than I suggest you go back and really think hard about the items you listed and see if you can come up with a few more that move you.

1. _____

2. _____

3. _____

4. _____

5. _____

Now I want you to circle 1, 2 or 3 that you are going to focus on for this first time through the exercise. You will come back to these in the next activity.

» ACTIVITY » WHO, WHAT, WHERE AND WHEN

In this simple, 3-minute activity, let's take the 1-3 goals from the previous activity and make them as specific as possible.

Remember this is the who, what, where and when of your goal.

Your Goal #1: _____

The Specifics: _____

_____

Your Goal #2: _____

The Specifics: _____

_____

Your Goal #3: _____

The Specifics: _____

_____

» Activity » Making it A Breeze to Succeed with Your Invincible Health and Fitness Goals

This is a worksheet where you can bring home your goals and truly make them a breeze to succeed. In this activity, I want you to figure out why you want to accomplish your goal.

So get at it and bring these goals closer to home now and do them with energy and vibrancy! You will find that success also requires you to be excited about your goals!

Fitness and Health Goal #1:

_____

_____

My Purpose for achieving it:

_____

_____

_____

_____

Fitness and Health Goal #2:

_____

_____

My Purpose for achieving it:

_____

_____

_____

_____

Fitness and Health Goal #3:

_____

_____

My Purpose for achieving it:

_____

_____

_____

_____

On the website, I've included some incredible tips on what you need to do to make these goals stick like glue in your conscious mind. Visit http://www.LiveAwesome.com/book to learn these easy and effective tips.

Mind Workout Step #8: How to Absolutely and Positively KNOW You Will Get the Health and Fitness Results You Desire

» Action » Make Your Image Collage

> A competitive world has two possibilities for you: you can lose or, if you want to win, you can change. — Lester C. Thurow

Mankind has known the power of visualization for thousands of years.

Have you ever seen pictures of cave drawings? You know, the ones where the hunter chases after the buffalo and then is drawn jumping around with his spear in victory in the last picture of the sequence? These guys knew how to motivate themselves!

Athletes do the same. They keep pictures of successful people in their lockers and they hang posters of their heroes. By doing this, they are using visual goals on their paths to success.

So what makes you any different? ABSOLUTELY NOTHING. If you start to make these goals come alive through pictures, then you start achieving them before you even lift one finger to exercise!

Think about how you would feel if you were running in a race and you came around a bend or up over a hill and saw the finish line up ahead. What would you do? You speed up, right? Why? Because now your goals are right there in front of you. It is a visual fact and it is absolutely and fantastically real.

This is the purpose of the image collage or mind map. The image collage—the final step to succeeding with your fitness and health goals— projects your goals visually, so you can see them every day and know that you are moving toward that finish line of fantastic fitness and absolute energy.

An image collage is a collage, just like the ones you might have done in grade school. Except this time it is a serious way to accomplish your goals.

To make one all you need to do is find a 8.5 X 11 sheet of paper (or larger if you like!), grab a bunch of old magazines and then start cutting out different pictures and words that support the goals you've set!

This is a breeze to do for the creative. For the not so creative it is also a breeze because you don't need to worry how it looks... all you need to worry about is if all your goals are represented in the form of images and words.

I've seen elaborate image collages with frills and borders and hand drawn pictures and I've seen collages with just a few cut out pictures and words. They both work just as well.

I have image collages for just about everything. Personal goals, business goals, fitness goals, you name it. They are posted for me to see so when I try to talk myself out of a workout or a decision, I can walk up to them and see my goals.

When you don't have these images, your conscious mind gets tricky with you and tells you all these things that might not be in your best interest like: We are feeling a little too tired or that show is on TV, let's watch that instead.

 With an image collage, you will have the power to convince your conscious mind that you are moving toward something of greater value—your health—than what seems to be more important at that particular moment.

» ACTIVITY » MAKING YOUR SUCCESS IMAGE COLLAGE

You want to hear something that will really get you excited about doing these collages?! I accomplish 80-90% of EVERY thing pictured on my image collages. I still find it incredible! Almost everything I put into image form happens!

You may ask what about the other 10-20%. The other 10-20% are by no means failures. Inevitably, these are always the things that I didn't really want and the things that I was doing not necessarily for myself. These are things that I didn't want in the first place!

To start your image collage you only need a few items:

1. An 8.5 X 11 piece of paper. (Just normal letter sized.)
2. Some old or new magazines. (Depending on your budget!)
3. Scissors.
4. Tape or glue
5. About an hour!

That's it. When you are making this collage here are some guidelines I'd like you to follow.

Make sure everything you put on the paper is positive. I only want you to put images that support your goals.

Make sure you are thinking about your goals and how it will feel to complete them and how wonderful that success will be!

You might want to do this activity with a spouse or a friend because it is a fun exercise to share with the people that you love!

Where do you put your Image Collage?

As long as you can see it everyday, it doesn't matter where. Some people put it on their closet door, others on their bathroom mirror… I put most of mine on the refrigerator. Just as long as you can see it regularly, then you will start achieving your goals.

For absolute best results put them everywhere… particularly where you see them all the time. Here are some more examples:

- On a door you enter and exit through everyday.
- By your bedroom light switch.
- Near the face of your alarm clock.
- By the interior handle of your car door.
- Next to your computer keyboard or monitor.
- Make a small copy and put it in your wallet.
- On the microwave door.
- By the telephone.
- In the shower stall.

You may feel uncomfortable putting these everywhere because your friends and family might make fun of you or think you are a quack.

If so, I'd like to pose this question to you: Would you rather be made fun of and in the best shape of your life, or stay where you are, just to avoid some harmless harassment?

One more secret about the Image Collage:

YOU HAVE TO SHARE IT WITH OTHERS. You have to tell people about your goals; because when you do you begin to attract whatever it is that will help you achieve them.

To see a few examples of image collages and get a better idea of what yours should look like, visit http://www.LiveAwesome.com/book.

The sun's light, diffused, is gentle warmth; directed through a magnifying glass in a certain way, it is incendiary.

— Maxwell Maltz, M.D.

QUICK FACT:

AT LEAST 74,868,455 (MILLION) AMERICANS WILL PARTICIPATE IN ABSOLUTELY NO LEISURE TIME ACTIVITY THIS YEAR. NOT EVEN AN AFTER DINNER WALK.

Statistics from www.cdc.gov and www.census.gov.

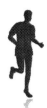 SECTION #3

THE 12 SIMPLE-TO-MAKE HEALTH AND FITNESS CHANGES YOU CAN MAKE TODAY TO START LOSING WEIGHT AND FEELING FANTASTIC IN DAYS!

Now that you are mentally prepared to reach your health and fitness goals with ease, here are the 12 simple steps to start achieving them today!

You can use this section just like the previous sections. Start in order and take action on each suggestion, or read the ones that interest you when you have the time.

Yes, I remember how busy you are... though most people seem to mysteriously have a little more available time if they've come this far. Starting to get it?

Again, I want to emphasize, if you do these steps in order and take action immediately after you read the chapter, your health and fitness will transform right before your eyes.

It doesn't matter if you try and try and try again, and fail.
It does matter if you try and fail, and fail to try again.
— Charles Kettering

THE BUSY PERSON'S SOLUTION #1: STOP SITTING AROUND LIKE A SLAB OF MEAT

» ACTION » START MOVING

Your first assignment is simple. Start moving.

Get up from your computer, your TV, from reading this book and take your first step forward. You're not too busy to take some "action" time.

There are no rules here. I don't care what you do and I don't care how long you do it for. You can swing your arms around like mad or take a walk in the park. Just start to get your systems moving.

I find that the people who succeed the most, just get up and go.

There are three exercises that I think are the absolute best for you. They work for me, my clients and many others. Best of all, they are very cheap and very easy.

Here they are:

- Walking
- Running
- Yoga

If you haven't taken to any of them in the past, I'd like you to give each activity another shot.

This doesn't mean go out and run six miles like you did in high school. It means take a walk. If that's too easy then start by walking and if you feel like running, jog for a minute, then slow down when it gets to be too much.

 Walking is the Most Efficient Fat Burning Exercise EVER!

Simpler is better.

We are meant to walk. We've been walking for thousands and thousands of years and as far as I know we haven't started evolving away from the heel-toe type transportation.

If you walk, you will lose weight. Walking brings your heart rate into a fat burning zone, which means you are using fat as fuel. This is great news for anyone who needs to burn anywhere from 5 to 500 pounds.

 I've come across many people who've lost a bunch of weight on their own. I'd say about 80-90% say that they just started walking—no free weights, no trainers, no cross trainers, just a pair of shoes and a road, sidewalk, or trail.

When you walk, you are generally in a fat-burning metabolic zone. This means that your body is using the by-products of fat synthesis as a fuel. You can know you're in a fat-burning metabolic zone if your heart is beating steadily and you're able to carry on a conversation easily while you're walking.

Walking at a fat burning mode, not only burns fat, but it also releases fat soluble vitamins into your blood stream—which have been stored in your adipose tissue (fat cells). Some of these fat soluble vitamins are powerful anti-oxidants. These anti-oxidants will neutralize the free radicals—cells damaged by activity through oxidation—you naturally create when you exercise. Talk about a well-oiled machine! This is one reason you feel great after a brisk walk.

So before anything else, make walking your priority. Walk after dinner, walk when you get up, walk up the stairs, walk down the stairs, walk to the store, walk back, walk everywhere.

By doing so, you'll strengthen your heart and your circulation, your muscles, your mind and your mood.

How to Walk More During the Day

Here are a few tips that will help you get more walking out of your waking hours!

- Walk at the park before or after work.
- Take a lunch break walk.
- Get off the subway or bus a stop or two earlier.
- Walk the stairs.
- Don't take the cab for less than 10-20 blocks. (Depending on the city or town you're in!)
- Walk the perimeter of your work building (inside or out).
- Walk at the mall.
- Take more walk breaks at work. (Walk to the water cooler more often, use a bathroom that is farther away.)
- If you work at home, walk to the mailbox and then down the street and back.

There are thousands of ways to walk more and you just need to get creative. City dwellers, suburbanites, and country folk all face different challenges. Distance, no sidewalks, the car culture, or time, are just a few. Regardless, getting more motion into your day is a success for any one of these people.

A Note on Running

One major reason most people don't like running is because they're doing it too fast. Slow down, don't get out of breath and you'll realize how fantastic it really is.

Running in a fat-burning zone should be just as easy as walking. You should not be out of breath and you should also be able to carry on a conversation. (See "The Busy Person's Solution #11: Use Your Heart as Your Guide and Save a Boatload of Time" for a more detailed explanation of your Fat-Burning Heart Rate and how to determine what works for you.)

If your knees are shot and you have other assorted aches and pains, don't run. Just walk. Walking is the most efficient exercise out there. Even if you've never exercised before in your life, you know how to walk. Do it!

A Note on Yoga

 Yoga is fantastic because it strengthens, stretches, and burns fat all at the same time. It is an extremely efficient practice for the busy person.

It's cheap to do also. Get a $10 mat, a $25 video and you're ready to go.

Let me be frank, if you give me the excuse that you still won't be able to find the time to do it, you need to go back and do a better job of assessing your goals. If you're still thinking that way, your goals are not strong enough.

By chance if you do happen to go out and do one, two or all of these activities and continue to not like them, then do something else. Play soccer, basketball, go rowing, rent a kayak or just keep trying other things until you find something you absolutely enjoy.

You are meant to move. Your body naturally agrees with motion. You will find something. Do something—take action—and then decide what works for you.

» ACTIVITY » TAKE ACTION AND GET MOVING!

By now, you should be motivated to get moving. So now it's time for you to actually do something. (If you haven't already!)

These activities are so easy that it pains me to tell you that they are really all you need to do to get into shape!

You probably already know that you don't need to do anything dramatic to lose weight, but do you really believe that this is all it takes? I bet you don't. I didn't for years!

Here are a few ideas you can use to start up and take action:

- Put down this book and take a walk right now.
  (Why are you still reading?!?!)
- Find a local walking, running or hiking club and mark the meeting time in your calendar
- Visit a local yoga studio
- Get a new pair of shoes at the local running/walking store...
  avoid the big chain stores and super-stores.
  (Find out why @ http://www.LiveAwesome.com/book)
- Call a friend to see if they want to join you for a walk, run or yoga class.
- Find a local basketball, tennis, soccer, etc. club.
- If you don't have time for that walk... do a one minute stretch routine right now. (Touch your toes, roll your neck, and then stand up and twist at your hips)

The Busy Person's Solution #2: Eliminate These 11 Foods and Additives from Your Diet for Optimal Health

» Action » Clean Out Your Cabinets

Are these 11 foods really that bad?

Yes.

If you want to be in fantastic shape and want to be a health and fitness success you need to stop eating them. The people you see who look and feel great, don't eat these things. Neither should you.

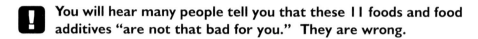 **You will hear many people tell you that these 11 foods and food additives "are not that bad for you." They are wrong.**

If you run into a person like this, ask them where they've received their information. They most likely will not be able to tell you.

As the ultimate test, look to see if they radiate good health and fantastic energy—if they don't I'm going to guess they have been moderately killing themselves by eating these foods.

This book is an easy way to achieve fantastic health and fitness. If you do everything here you will succeed. Don't listen to anyone who WANTS to be there. Listen to someone who IS there.

If you're still questioning whether or not you should eat a food on this list, here's one other way to look at it.

If just a few drops of cyanide can kill you, what else can?

1. Cigarettes and Nicotine

Duh.

2. Aspartame or any artificial sweetener.

You are better off eating sugar than putting poisons like aspartame in your body. If you eat it for diet or any purposes, think about this: The American Cancer Society found that those who used sweetener in their diets actually gained more weight than those who didn't!

Aspartame can cause cancer, lupus and M.S. Some symptoms of Aspartame poisoning are joint pain, diarrhea, depression, cramps, spasms, dizziness, shooting pains, seizures and numbness in your legs.

If you eat too much aspartame you can die.

This is a synthetic product that has no equivalent in nature. Your body was never meant to have it. Why take the risk?

3. High Fructose Corn Syrup

High fructose corn syrup (HFCS), made from cornstarch, became prevalent in our foods in the 1970s when the food industry found that it was sweeter and cheaper than regular table sugar (sucrose).

This highly processed sugar is linked to weight gain and diabetes and is more likely to be turned to fat by the body than any of the other sugars.

This sugar is added to many processed foods and even the foods that say "Fat Free." Here is a popular—but not exclusive—list:

- Soft Drinks
- Fruit Juices
- Baked Goods
- Canned Fruit
- Dairy Products
- Cookies
- Gum
- Jams and Jellies
- Salad Dressings

HFCS also raises your triglyceride levels. High levels are linked to heart disease as well as general deteriorating health.

This processed food, just like the others on this list, is a poison and you cannot continue to be confused by the studies that say it is good for you.

HFCS might have one or two good qualities—it is cheap and makes things taste good—but that isn't enough reason to put it in our food and make us fat!

4. Hydrogenated Oils (Trans Fats) and Partially Hydrogenated Oils

The process of hydrogenation started in the 1950s to extend packed food shelf life. Hydrogenation is the process of heating oil and passing hydrogen bubbles through it. The fatty acids in the oil then acquire some of the hydrogen, which makes it denser. If you fully hydrogenate, you create a solid (a fat) out of the oil. But if you stop part way, you get a semi-solid partially hydrogenated oil that has a consistency like butter, but much cheaper.

These fats also called, trans-fats, disguise themselves as regular fats, and build up in your arteries. The difference is that they don't do the same job as the regular fats in your body do, so instead of escorting poisons and toxins to your liver and protecting your body, they hang around, build on your arteries and cause heart disease and arteriosclerosis.

Trans-fats are poisons. They interfere with the metabolic process by taking the place of a natural substance (good fats) that performs a critical function. Your body has no defense against them.

And get this…

 Many European countries have either BANNED or have set dates for ELIMINATION of hydrogenated oils in foods!

Hydrogenated oils are found in almost all packaged foods. Take a look at the ingredients the next time you are at the grocery store and you will see just how prevalent these are in the foods you eat. Here's a list of products that contain them:

Foods Almost Always Made With Hydrogenated Oils
- Cake mixes, biscuit, pancake and cornbread mixes, frostings
- Cakes, cookies, muffins, pies, donuts
- Crackers
- Peanut butter (except fresh-ground)
- Frozen entrees and meals
- Frozen bakery products, toaster pastries, waffles, pancakes
- Most prepared frozen meats and fish (such as fish sticks)
- French fries
- Whipped toppings
- Margarines, shortening
- Instant mashed potatoes
- Taco shells
- Cocoa mix
- Microwave popcorn

Many Brands of these Foods are Made with Partially Hydrogenated Oils
- Breakfast cereals
- Corn chips, potato chips
- Frozen pizza, frozen burritos, most frozen snack foods
- Low-fat ice creams
- Noodle soup cups
- Bread
- Pasta mixes
- Sauce mixes

Read The Labels! And Don't Buy Them!

AUTHOR's NOTE: Watch out for this new trick! I recently saw a bag of Cheetos that was advertising "0 Grams of Trans Fat" on the front of the bag. Skeptical, I took a look at the ingredients and saw that, in fact, partially hydrogenated oil was one of the ingredients. After a double take, I went home to see how they could possibly get away with this.

According to the FDA, "if the serving contains less than 0.5 gram [of trans fat], the content, when declared, shall be expressed as zero."

So if those Cheetos contain 0.4 grams per serving and you eat four or five servings, (this is not uncommon practice!) you have just consumed 1.6-2.0 grams of trans fat, despite the fact that the front and the back label of the package claims that the product contains zero grams of trans fat per serving!

Believe me when I say this: you're blatantly being tricked by marketers everyday.

5. Coffee

Cringe....

Yes, coffee contains caffeine--a diuretic--that increases the frequency of urination which causes dehydration. It keeps you awake, elevates your heart rate, blood pressure and increases the secretion of acid into your stomach... blah, blah, blah.

What concerns me most is that coffee puts stress on your adrenal system. This translates to more stress. Aren't you under enough stress already?

Coffee drinkers tend to use the drink as a pick-me-up, but what happens is that it becomes a drag-me-down, because the body, while it experiences a short caffeine buzz, drops to a lower energy level when the high wears off. At this lover level, you're not only feeling down, but you're burning your sugar stores. This creates sugar cravings. Heard of coffee and doughnuts?

When I stopped drinking coffee and switched to herbal teas in the morning, I found I could hop out of bed and never think twice about having a cup of coffee.

To get off coffee, here's my solution. Stop drinking it for 10 days. After you've experienced the headaches, the shaking, and have sweat through every waking hour of those 10 days without your coffee, on the 11th day drink 4 cups in the morning in a 1-hour time frame. (Be sure you're by a toilet.)

I guarantee you'll never want to drink it again. The stuff is poison and it kills your energy levels!

6. Soda

Soda is simply sugar. I can't tell you how many people I've known who quit drinking soda shed a bunch of weight. I don't mean 1-2 pounds, I mean 10-15. There are 250 calories in a 20-oz bottle of Coke. Not to mention there is caffeine!

Take the effects of caffeine and add them to a sugar overload and you have one unhealthy body. Do you drink soda and coffee?! If so, and you want more energy, I will tell you right now that dropping those two poisonous habits will improve your daily stamina by 100%!

What about diet soda? I've already told you about aspartame.

7. Fast Food

No Whoppers, No Big Macs, No NOTHING. These foods are stuffed with hydrogenated oils, artificial flavors, saturated fats, and sugars... this is poison central. Don't eat it! It makes you tired, fat and sick. These foods are engineered to make you want more and feel lousy.

Don't eat quasi-fast food either. These include chains like Chili's, Olive Garden, Perkin's and the hundreds of others along our major thoroughfares and interstate exits. They get their foods from some of the same sources that the easily identifiable fast food joints use. It's the same stuff, just a little prettier and more expensive.

If you travel or are on the road a lot, pack a bunch of fresh fruit and vegetables (mini carrots, celery, etc.) so you can snack while you're driving. If you absolutely want some carbs, buy a bag of veggie chips or something to crunch on. Also, bring a ton of water so you can stay hydrated and awake.

8. "Artificial Flavors"

Artificial Flavors are chemicals that are put in our foods to add flavor to food products that are so over processed that they no longer have any taste at all.

It's disgusting and we're buying into it every time we go to the supermarket.

Most artificial additives are made from derivatives of crude oil that are chemically altered to produce a synthetic substance. You can see why this might be a health concern.

This is not food.

There are health effects associated with artificial additives and flavors and what's worse is that they are added most to the foods that already have had their nutrients stripped from them by artificial pesticides and fertilizers. Here are some to watch out for.

Artificial Colors (listed on labels as F D & C colors, or as a specific color such as Yellow #5): These are made from coal-tar and have been shown to cause cancer in laboratory animals. Yum.

BHA and BHT: These are also made from coal-tar and have been linked to hyperactive behavior in children. They are on the FDA's GRAS list (Generally Recognized As Safe).

EDTA (ethylenediamine tetraacetic acid): This synthetic chemical is made from minerals, is irritating to the skin and can cause allergic reactions. It also can cause kidney damage. Funny thing is, even though it's on the FDA list for further study, it's still in our food.

Nitrates and Nitrites: Nitrates and Nitrites are made from mineral salts. These are known to cause cancer in animals. They are added to most pork, especially processed meats, as well as some other meat, poultry, fish, and cheese.

Sulfites (sulfur dioxide, sodium sulfite, sodium and potassium bisulfite, sodium and potassium metabisulfite): These are made from sulfur and mineral salts. They can cause severe allergic reactions, including breathing difficulties, gastrointestinal disorders, unconsciousness, hives, and anaphylactic shock. Found in many processed foods and almost always in wine and beer.

One insidious trick the food industry uses to get around putting all these artificial ingredients on the label is this: they'll put an ingredient in a processed food, list it on the package, and then never break down the individual ingredients in that specific ingredient.

Here's an example:

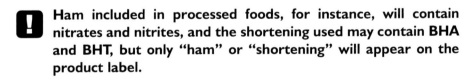 **Ham included in processed foods, for instance, will contain nitrates and nitrites, and the shortening used may contain BHA and BHT, but only "ham" or "shortening" will appear on the product label.**

9. "Natural Flavors" and "Spices"

Any package that says "Natural" on the front or the back generally means that the product does not contain any added "artificial" (having no counterpart in nature) additives, but it does not necessarily mean pesticides or other chemicals were not used in processing.

Your potato chips that say "natural" could be genetically altered, grown with pesticides, and cleaned with unfiltered water and still read "All Natural!"

What is scary is that natural flavors and spices are assumed to be OK.

But what is not OK is that any substance derived from something natural, no matter how dangerous it is, can be classified as a "natural flavoring." What's worse is that if a poisonous chemical is used to derive that flavoring, it can still be called "natural".

Many natural flavors are synthesized from Isoprene, which is a known carcinogen! Isoprene stays in the food… it doesn't just disappear!

Manufacturers also hide monosodium glutamate (MSG)—a flavoring which causes headaches and allergic reactions—in their "natural flavorings" or "spices" listings because it is derived from seaweed, a natural product. So clearly, being natural is not the same as being harmless.

 Tip: If you have migraines… stop eating foods with MSG… you might be surprised.

Here are some terms that often indicate hidden MSG additives:
• Malt extract
• Bouillon
• Broth
• Stock
• Flavoring
• Natural Flavoring
• Natural Beef or Chicken Flavoring
• Seasoning
• Spices

10. Irradiated Foods

Food irradiation is done by zapping food with a dosage of radiation. The X-rays are used to kill insects and bacteria, prevent sprouting, and slow rotting.

While the process does not make the food radioactive, the chemical structure of the food is altered and there are a number of animal studies that show negative health effects.

Some researchers suspect that a regular diet of irradiated food may cause leukemia, other forms of cancer, and kidney disease. The FDA says it's safe.

When you hear that, I want you to think about other things that were apparently safe… such as cigarette smoking, pesticides, asbestos and CFCs. Each of these at one time was classified as safe.

The FDA claims irradiation of food is safe and has already authorized the irradiation of fruits, vegetables, pork, chicken, herbs, spices, teas, and seeds. Spices are the most widely irradiated food in the United States.

You can avoid irradiation by buying 100% organic spices and foods.

NOTE: Avoid the microwave as well. This type of irradiation affects the chemistry of foods by activating the water molecules inside. If cooking does some damage to enzymes and foods, then microwaving is the equivalent to a nuclear blast, leaving everything once living lifeless and wilted.

11. Chemicals

This is the catch-all...

As a general rule, anything that's longer than 15 letters, you can't pronounce and is hyphenated is generally not good for you.

For information on how to quit smoking, aspartame, food poisons, reading food labels and more, please visit my website @ www.LiveAwesome.com/book.

» ACTIVITY » CABINET CLEANING 101

This activity is easier than you think!

I want you to go into your cabinet and your refrigerator and take a look at the foods that are there. Look at the back of the labels. If you see any of the foods or additives I mentioned, I'd like you to put them on the counter. Do the same for the refrigerated goods and frozen goods.

Once everything is separated... foods with toxins on the counter and foods with no toxins still in the fridge or the panty, I want you to arrange them all. Put the good foods on one side of the refrigerator and pantry and the bad foods on the other. I'm not asking you to throw anything away... just separate them!

I want you to be aware of the amount of products that you have in your house that can be poisoning your body.

I want you to leave them separated and every time you go into the cabinet or the fridge think about what they are doing to your body when you ingest them.

Think about how the poisons are depriving you of your energy every time you open up the refrigerator or the pantry.

Think about how awful the food industry is to be putting these poisons in your food just to deepen their pockets.

If you do this a few times a day, I guarantee after 4-5 days you'll start to rethink your stance on how you should eat and how much healthier you can be by eating the right foods that fuel your body with an abundance of energy.

 Remember your food is affecting your ability to live an energized and vibrant life. Don't let it stop you!

PHENOMENAL HEALTH AND FITNESS SECRET
TREAT CARBOHYDRATES LIKE THE SUGARS THEY REALLY ARE

Carbohydrates are sugars. Treat them that way.

That doesn't mean they are bad or good. You just need to change your perspective on them.

The bread may not taste sweet, but it's loaded with sugar energy. Once you start chewing, your saliva turns carbohydrates into sugar. That's where your cravings begin.

The carbohydrate—now sugar—then goes into your bloodstream. If there's already enough sugar in the blood (blood sugar) then the pancreas secretes insulin to lower blood sugar. The insulin turns this sugar into fat and stores it for later.

After this process runs its course, your blood sugar is left significantly lower and you actually start craving more sugar (breads, carbohydrates) because you now have low blood sugar levels.

Then, again, bread goes in, blood sugar goes up, insulin is released and you continue to get fat.

! **Treat breads and pastas like the sugars they really are and you'll lose weight quickly. Look at your plate of pasta and loaf of bread like a piece of cake. They're both filled with sugars. Would you eat cake every meal?**

No. So apply the same principle to pastas and breads. Eat them in extreme moderation and eat only whole grains.

Whole grains are a better choice because, unlike white or processed grains, they still have many of their nutrients intact. When you eat a whole grain, there are complementary minerals (chromium is one in particular) that help regulate your body's reaction to the sugar in the grain. These minerals don't allow the same rapid spike and drop in blood sugar that processed grains do, nor do they cause the same extreme surge of insulin in your blood stream.

THE BUSY PERSON'S SOLUTION #3: STOP EATING LIKE A JAPANESE COMPETITIVE EATER!

» ACTION » BE CONSCIOUS OF YOUR EATING

Smaller is better when it comes to portion sizes.

I went to the Annual Hot Dog Eating Contest in Coney Island when I lived in Brooklyn. There were about 20 contestants from all over the world competing to see how many hot dogs (with buns) they could stuff in their throats in a given time. The winner from Japan managed to stuff over 50 hot dogs down his throat in a matter of minutes! Those guys could definitely use a lesson on portion control.

I was always taught to finish everything on my plate. My mother would tell me that I'd have to do so in order to leave the table or if I wanted dessert. There were times when I forced it down just to get up from the table. My brother was even more stubborn. I can remember the whole family leaving the table to leave him leaning over a serving of green beans that he was just too full to put down.

For my brother and me—and I'm sure for most of you—this was a powerful and lasting lesson in overeating. There are still times when I need to take control over my portion size, because that was so deeply ingrained in my head at such a young age.

Here's How to Control Your Portion Size with Ease:

1. Serve your own plate.

If you let someone else serve you (particularly an Italian mother) you are going to get too much. If you are aware of your food intake and how hungry you are, you will actually put just the right amount of food on your plate.

2. Don't Take Seconds.

In an hour or so if you are still hungry, have some more.

3. Eat Small Snacks During the Day.

I have a fresh juice or different snacks during the day to keep my energy up, so when it comes to mealtime, I don't pack in a turkey dinner for a family of five.

4. Eat More Vegetables than Meat.

This is simple plate geometry. Your plate should have about 2/3 vegetables and no more than 1/3 anything else. Steak should not be the centerpiece. This allows you to fill up on vegetables, fibers and a small amount of carbohydrates—not meat.

5. Eat Your Salad First.

Eat the salad first. You will fill up quicker and eat smaller portions!

6. Chew!

You're not a pig, so don't eat like one! Take some time to breathe between bites. You'll eat less and feel better.

When you go out to dinner, take a moment to really look at the sizes of the portions. They are absolutely too big! Split your dinner in two and eat the other half for lunch. You will drop weight immediately.

» ACTIVITY » RECOGNIZING PATTERNS WITH A FOOD LOG

! **Food logs are *fantastic* tools to identify habits in your eating. Why? Because you forget what you eat.**

Think about what you ate 4 days ago for dinner. Remember? I don't either!

What the food log can do is identify foods you eat too much of, foods that are harmful to your body and how you felt when you ate those foods. So if you are the type of person who eats when you are sad, or tired, or watching TV... you now have a record of it and can see your eating habit patterns.

You're going to do this for 3 days. Make copies if you need more lines!

Here are the rules:

1. Using the sheet I've provided, record everything you eat. This should include foods and beverages eaten at meals and snacks. Plus everything you added to them... salt, creamer, sugar, Equal—all of it!
2. Record carefully how the food was prepared. Be as descriptive as possible (e.g., fried in corn oil, broiled in margarine).
3. Be sure to indicate the amount of food eaten. Serving size is very important! Use cups, ounces, tablespoons, teaspoons for measurements.
4. Provide brand names and labels for packaged foods.
5. For sandwiches, casseroles, soups and other recipes indicate the ingredients contained in the food. For example, a turkey sandwich might be described as 2 slices of whole wheat bread, 1 oz. of baked turkey breast without skin, 1 slice of tomato, 2 leaves of iceberg lettuce, 1 tablespoon of light mayonnaise.
6. Indicate where and with whom you were with when you ate. Also describe your feelings at the time – were you worried, content, lonely, stressed? (Be honest with yourself.)
7. Carry this form with you so that you can write down foods as they are eaten. Do not wait until the end of the day to record your food intake.

When you are done, you then can compare the foods you ate with the information I've given you here!!

You can also go to our website http://www.LiveAwesome.com/book and figure out how many calories and nutrients you are getting on a daily basis based on your food log!

THE BUSY PERSON'S SOLUTION FOOD LOG

Food/Drink (Include Serving Size and Brand)	Time You Ate	What You Were Feeling Before and After Eating (Anxious, Hungry, Tired, Bored, Etc.)	Location (Home, Work, Driving, Etc)
	:		
	:		
	:		
	:		
	:		
	:		
	:		
	:		
	:		
	:		
	:		
	:		
	:		
	:		
	:		
	:		
	:		
	:		
	:		
	:		
	:		
	:		
	:		
	:		
	:		

Keep this with you at ALL TIMES!

THE BUSY PERSON'S SOLUTION #4: STOCK UP ON THESE FOODS LIKE A STORM WAS COMING

» ACTION » MAKE THESE FOODS STAPLES OF YOUR DIET.

If you introduce the foods in this chapter into your diet, your energy levels will skyrocket and your waistline will shorten!

Your food is what is used to form all the cells in your body. When you eat good food, your cells are good. When you eat bad food your cells are not healthy. This is a very simple concept that many people have ignored their ENTIRE LIFE!

I want to use the shower analogy again. Americans always find the time to shower.

Got to be somewhere in 20 minutes? No problem… hop in the shower for 5, leave in 8.

Those of you who take 3 hours… No problem. Wake up at 3:30 to be there by 9:00? No sweat.

No matter what, there's always time. Why is it not the same with the way we eat? We're all clean on the outside, but inside we're dirty as a chicken coup.

What if I told you that you should consider washing your body with antifreeze not soap? Wouldn't even think about it, right? You can find some of the same chemicals that wash our windshields and keep our car fluids from freezing in the ice creams that you buy in the supermarket!

How about brushing your teeth with pesticides? Pretty nauseating. Well, everyday Americans eat non-organic vegetables that are not only showered in pesticides, but grow in the ground that has been contaminated for years!

What I'm saying is this… In order for you to achieve and maintain your best fitness and health, you need to refine your fuel. Would you think about putting low grade gas in a brand new Ferrari? No WAY! You want the best for that engine, so now let me tell you about the best fuel for your engine— your body!

So what should you eat?

Live Foods

! **The best foods you can eat are fresh, organically grown, uncooked foods.**

The reason is because their chemistry has not been changed by cooking, pesticides or any other chemical additive. Your diet should consist of more raw foods than cooked if you want to have the most energy. Why? Because the cells in these foods are still living. They contain complete nutrients and enzymes that your body needs for maximum and optimal health.

If you have an onion in the pantry for too long it starts to grow! Those living enzymes, the same ones that make that onion grow are what you want to eat.

Another great thing about raw food is that nature has a fantastic way of putting complimentary nutrients together so they can work together on absorption. So you'll find the right amount of magnesium with calcium and vitamin D in a whole, raw food. You can't get that in most supplements. Most supplements can't imitate nature like this. With raw foods, it's what nature intended.

Now wait, please don't panic... you can still cook foods, cooking vegetables is much better than eating none at all, but make sure you bring more raw foods into your diet.

 The more raw foods you eat, the more life energy you will have.

Do it, you'll feel great and you'll make it a staple of your diet.

Good Fats

You need good fats. Olive oil, Flax Seed Oil, Avocado, Fish Oils, Udo's Oil, Raw Coconut Oil, Raw Hemp Seed, and Some nuts and seeds (almonds, sunflower seeds, brazil nuts, hazelnuts, pumpkin seeds).

These support cell membrane development, which supports flow of fluids, fats, nutrients and cells through your body. (Bad fats are the "frieds", margarine, and animal fats.)

Take some Omega 3 Oils. Put them on your salad, take them in pills... whatever you like, just get them in your body and everything will start to flow better.

Eating the right foods is all about efficiency. Once your body is flowing then you eliminate things right away and the toxins will no longer set up shop in your organs, blood or bones.

There's a bunch of talk about what omega-3 fats are better for different people. Go out and try them and see how they work for you. Don't get caught up in the hype.

Take action. Get results.

Organic Foods:

> Buy organic.
>
> I have a list of over 100 foods and the pesticides that are in them that will make you think differently about non-organic foods. The list was put out by the FDA. If this doesn't convince you, I don't know what will.
>
> *It is way to long to include here…*
>
> *You can find it on my site @ http://www.LiveAwesome.com/book.*
>
> *Look for "FDA Whole Food Study"*

There are two prevalent reasons why people don't eat organic foods.

1. "They are too expensive."

Yes, organics are a little more expensive. Think of this expense as an insurance premium. You most likely pay less for your medications and co-pays—if any—when you're 45 if you don't have any known health conditions caused by pesticides in your food.

Stop making your food purchases based on price. You are making a huge mistake.

If I were selling two cars, one, that looks great with a great engine for $4000 and, the other, the same model that is in exactly the same shape, but without an engine, working radio and no transmission, for $3800, which one would you buy?

You'd buy the one that works right? Of, course. There's no sense in buying the car that needs more components when there's one that already has them. So wouldn't you do the same with your food?

Chances are, if your buying food based on the week's special, you're getting the car without the engine, radio and transmission. So you're paying pennies less, but you're getting robbed!

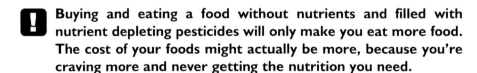 **Buying and eating a food without nutrients and filled with nutrient depleting pesticides will only make you eat more food. The cost of your foods might actually be more, because you're craving more and never getting the nutrition you need.**

Also, if more people buy organics, the price WILL go down. It already has since the late 1990's. This is the simple economics of supply and demand.

2. "It doesn't matter if it is organic or not."

Say you asked me for an apple and I grabbed one from the fruit basket and sprayed some Raid on it, then gave it to you. Would you eat it?

What if I took that same apple with Raid all over it and washed it in the sink—then gave it to you. Would you eat it then? Probably not. Pesticides are real and they are poisons.

Take a look at the list I mentioned above from the FDA. There are still residues of DDT (a dangerous pesticide banned decades ago) in our vegetables and foods. If you still disagree, then you're on your own.

Here is a short list of some of the healthiest foods that you can find at the grocery store:

Vegetables and Root Vegetables (Organic): Asparagus, Avocado, Bell peppers, Broccoli, Brussels Sprouts, Cabbage, Cauliflower, Celery, Collard Greens, Cucumber, Dandelion Greens, Eggplant, Fennel, Garlic, Green beans, Green peas, Kale, Leeks, Mushrooms (Shiitake and Crimini), Mustard Greens, Olives, Onions, Parsley, Romaine Lettuce, Sea Vegetables, Spinach, Squash, Swiss Chard, Tomato, Turnip Greens, Beets, Carrots, Sweet Potatoes, Yams.

Fish & Seafood (Wild Caught): Cod, Halibut, Salmon, Snapper, Tilapia, Tuna, Yellowfin

Fruits (Organic): Apple, Apricot, Banana, Blackberries, Blueberries, Cherries, Fig, Grapefruit, Grapes, Kiwi fruit, Lemon and Limes, Orange, Papaya, Pears, Pineapple, Plantains, Plum, Prunes, Raisins, Raspberries, Strawberries, Watermelon.

Beans & Legumes (Organic): Black Beans, Peas, Garbanzo Beans, Kidney Beans, Lentils, Lima Beans, Navy Beans, Pinto Beans, Tempeh, Tofu

Poultry & Lean Meats (Organic and Naturally Fed): Beef, Lamb, Turkey, Venison

Nuts & Seeds (Raw): Almonds, Flaxseeds, Olive Oil, Pumpkin Seeds, Sesame Seeds, Sunflower Seeds, Walnuts, Cashews, Hemp Seeds, Brazil Nuts.

Grains (Organic): Barley, Buckwheat, Cous Cous, Millet, Oats, Quinoa, Brown Rice, Rye, Spelt, Wheat

Spices & Herbs (Organic, Non-Irradiated): Basil, Cayenne Pepper, Red Chili Pepper, Cilantro, Cinnamon, Cloves, Coriander Seeds, Cardamom, Cumin Seeds, Dill Weed, Ginger, Mint, Mustard Seeds, Oregano, Parsley, Peppermint Leaves, Rosemary, Sage, Thyme, Turmeric

Natural Sweeteners: Raw Cane juice, Raw Honey, Raw Maple syrup

» ACTIVITY » GO SHOPPING!

Here's your mission.

I want you to pick twenty of the foods on the above list… or you can use my suggestions and go out and buy the foods I've listed below.

Try them. You don't have to like all of them. My intention is to open up your palate to some different options. We get stuck. Here's your opportunity to get "un-stuck" and get very healthy!

Shopping List (All vegetables should be Organic):

- Carrots
- Kale
- Collard Greens
- Raw Beets (Not Pickled)
- Green Cabbage
- Parsley
- Cilantro
- Blueberries
- Cherries
- Apples

- Wild Caught Salmon
- Quinoa
- Brown Rice
- Dried Prunes
- Raw Sunflower Seeds
- Raw Pumpkin Seeds
- Raw Almonds
- Raw Almond Butter
- Raw Honey
- Raw Brazil Nuts

Don't know how to prepare any of these foods?
Visit http://www.LiveAwesome.com/book for a bunch of quick, healthy and energy boasting recipes!

Phenomenal Health and Fitness Secret
Eat Highly Mineralized Meals and Superfoods and You'll Never Gain Another Pound

Forget grams of protein, grams of fat, and grams of carbohydrates for a minute.

I want you to think about minerals and vitamins. If you eat synthetically enriched, processed grains; mineral-poor, corn-fed cattle; and vegetables grown in mineral depleted soils, you can get all the carbohydrates, fats and proteins you'll ever need.

What you won't get is the nutrients to support your body's functions.

Highly mineralized foods are the next health food wave—after this wave of organics—and they are for good reason. Your body needs good minerals and vitamins for everything from muscle-firing to brain functioning.

Our soils are depleted of minerals. The foods we are getting now are not as rich in minerals as they were 50 years ago due to over-use of farmland, synthetic fertilizers and hybrid or modified plant species. As of 2002, the JAMA reversed its 30 year position on supplementation—stating that taking mineral and vitamin supplements is now necessary due to poor mineral content in our soils.

There are a few ways to get more minerals. You can supplement your diet with good organic vitamins and minerals, you can juice fresh organic vegetables and fruits, and one of my favorite, is eating specific superfoods—whole foods that have extraordinary vitamin and mineral content.

These are all good techniques and I recommend you try them and see which one—or combination—works best for you.

If you're curious about what these superfoods are and where you can get them, turn the page and read on...

THE BUSY PERSON'S SOLUTION #5: BUY AND EAT THESE 7 SECRET FOODS THAT ONLY THE HEALTHIEST PEOPLE IN THE WORLD KNOW ABOUT!

» ACTION » ADD THESE SUPERFOODS TO YOUR DIET

Have you heard the buzz about superfoods?

If you haven't, the talk around the health and fitness world is that there are specific foods that give you more bang for your buck than others.

There is some mystique about that isn't there? Imagine a food—or a group of foods—that alone can elevate moods, enrich your body with almost hundreds of minerals and taste great all at the same time?

These foods are not just the "ordinary" superfoods like the cherry, the avocado or extra virgin olive oil. These foods are from the corners of the world and they will pack a super punch into your everyday diet.

Superfood #1: Cacao (Raw Chocolate)

Want more energy? Try some raw chocolate.

Raw chocolate is among the most powerful sources of magnesium on the planet. Not only does magnesium help with alertness and activity, it also helps elevate your mood.

Magnesium is one of the most deficient minerals in the human body. Depending on where you find your studies 60-80% of Americans are deficient in magnesium. No wonder we're sluggish, agitated and stressed!

Cooked chocolate does not possess all the fantastic health benefits as raw chocolate. So please don't use this as an excuse to stock up on chocolate bars and kisses! Your chocolate candy does not have the same composition as it does when it's raw. The raw version still has many nutrients and minerals in their natural composition. Your cooked candy bar does not. There actually is very little cacao in processed chocolate.

Raw chocolate also contains naturally occurring tryptophan—an essential amino acid—which helps naturally produce serotonin in your body. This is great news for those who need an emotional boost.

You can buy raw chocolate in the shell (it is a seed), but it's easiest if you buy it without.

Since the cacao bean is actually fairly bitter, it is best to mix it with various other superfoods—pumpkin seeds, goji berries—for a super, power-packed, nutrient-rich dry snack that will get you through even the toughest days.

Superfood #2: Goji Berries

Move over carrot.

This little, bright red berry from China is one of the most potent sources of beta-carotene. Beta-carotene is an anti-oxidant that can stop cell oxidation—or the spread of free-radicals. Beta carotene may also help prevent certain cancers, such as lung and prostate cancer.

Goji berries are also a good source of vitamin C which also is a fantastic anti-oxidant. Goji berries also contain 18 amino acids and over 21 minerals which give them a serious power-punch to anyone's system. In addition, goji berries help stimulate your body's natural human growth hormone which is critical in anti-aging and longevity.

You can only get dried goji berries in the US, so don't expect to find them in any produce section. Some health food stores will carry them, but you're best bet is online.

Goji berries make for a fantastic snack—eat them just like you would raisins—to add to your superfood arsenal and are a great addition to any herbal tea.

Superfood #3: Maca

Maca is a Peruvian root powder that is used to increase strength and vitality. It has more mineral content than potatoes and carrots—loaded with iron, magnesium, calcium, potassium, and iodine.

The Peruvians and many others claim Maca can help fight depression, help with anemia and improve overall memory and vitality.

This powerful food is also a libido stimulant and will help stimulate the thyroid!

Maca powder is best taken mixed with warm water in a tea. Maca has a strong taste which can be softened with goji berries or honey.

Superfood #4: Raw Honey

I'm not talking about the honey in the little bear. I'm talking real, unprocessed, raw honey.

Raw honey contains enzymes, phytonutrients, resins and propolis—bee glue. This unique combination of properties makes it versatile not only as a food, but as an anti-bacterial agent.

As a food, raw honey can raise antioxidant levels in the body, restore muscle glycogen after a workout and help lower cholesterol and the risk of certain cancers—honey does not cause acidity in the body which can be a contributing factor to some cancers. As a topical substance, it can decrease infection and work just as well as alcohol solutions. You can use raw honey as a sweetener, put some in your teas or your water, or just have a small spoonful for a quick pick me up.

(Be sure not to heat it to a high temperature. Heat will destroy many of its best qualities.)

Local raw honey has also been used to treat seasonal allergies. A small serving a day can give some people relief from their allergies homeopathically.

Superfood #5: Spirulina

This superfood (and the next) might scare some people off, but don't compromise your health by not trying these two foods!

The first, spirulina, is an algae that has high vegetable protein content, is high in B-12 vitamins and Gamma Linolenic Acid (GLA).

GLA and Vitamin B-12 are connected to mood, memory and general energy vitality. Many people believe that low B-12 levels for long periods of time is actually the cause of "old age" symptoms—fatigue, memory loss, confusion, etc.

Just because it is an algae doesn't mean that it's gross! The first time I tried it, I was surprised that it tasted so good.

Buy it in flakes and sprinkle it on your salads, add it to a smoothie, sauces, or soups.

Superfood #6: Sea Vegetables

Sea vegetables are grown in an environment full of minerals that our body needs for optimal health—the ocean. Ocean water has up to 92 minerals that can be absorbed by the plants growing in the sea.

This makes sea vegetables one of the most nutrient dense foods on the planet. Seaweed—compared to land vegetables—is one of the best vegetable sources of calcium, which is fantastic for muscle and bone development, strength, and growth.

Don't worry if the idea of eating seaweed grosses you out. Your health food store will have different seaweed granules that you can use as a salt substitute and you'll never know the difference.

Nori, dulce, and kelp are three of the most readily available sea vegetables.

Superfood #7: Pumpkin Seeds and More...

The raw pumpkin seed, just like the cacao bean, is another feel good food. It is a great source of magnesium and tryptophan. You can find this super-seed right in your backyard if you live in the Northeastern US!

Pumpkin seeds also are great sources of protein, fat and other essential minerals.

Other great seeds are hemp seed, flax seed and raw sunflower seeds. These all contain good fats and good protein for optimal health.

If you're eating a primarily vegetarian or vegan diet, be sure to add these seeds to your diet to get some good protein. If you're NOT a vegetarian or vegan, be sure to add these seeds to your diet to get some good protein (not a typo!).

They are great to add to salads as an extra garnish or great as a snack or mixed in with some other superfoods.

» ACTIVITY » GIVE THESE FOODS A SHOT AND SEE HOW THEY WORK FOR YOU!

This might be the easiest activity of all!

Go to the health food store or visit my site and try some of these foods! My advice is to start with the easiest first...

- Cacao
- Goji Berries
- Raw Honey
- Raw Pumpkin Seeds
- Raw Sunflower Seeds

Then eventually add the others into your everyday diet. Your body will thank you... I promise!

On the site, http://www.LiveAwesome.com/book, I've also provided a list of different ideas and recipes on how to get creative with these superfoods!

PHENOMENAL HEALTH AND FITNESS SECRET

THE ECONOMICS OF BREADS, CORN AND PASTAS HAVE PUT THEM ON OUR PLATES, NOT THEIR NUTRIENT VALUES.

Wheat flour, pastas, corn and breads are products of poor societies. The Egyptians used to pay their slaves in unleavened bread, because it was cheap and could keep them satiated. But the nutrient content of these breads was not rich, which led to the spread of diseases. You can trace this up through history.

I'm Italian. When my great-grandparents came from Italy they were poor and Roman Catholic. They had a bunch of kids and needed to feed them. Wheat flours, namely breads and pastas, were the cheapest food they could find.

So what did they eat? Bread and pasta. The food you're used to eating is not on your plate because it's healthy—it's there because of economic reasons.

In "Plan B: Rescuing a Planet Under Stress and a Civilization in Trouble," Lester Brown speaks about how the poorest billion people in the world are suffering from disease related to malnutrition. Their diet consists of at least 70% grains, which is the cheapest food available to them.

Corn is another food that has infiltrated our food supply in more ways than one. Food additives, such as, high fructose corn syrup (modified sugar), citric acid (a preservative), dextrin (a complex carbohydrate), caramel color, xanthan gum (a thickener), lecithin (an emulsifier that keeps fat and water from separating) and mono-, tri- and diglycerides (more emulsifiers) are all derived from corn! All of these additives are extremely prevalent in our food system. Just take a look at the labels on the back of the food you buy and I'm sure you'll be able to identify a few on almost any packaged product.

According to Michael Pollan author of "The Omnivore's Dilemma," a McDonald's cheeseburger is 52% corn. Milkshake? 78%. Your Soda? Besides the water, it's 100% corn.

Corn is not just in fast foods, it's in cereals, breads, frozen foods, salad dressings and baked goods. Why? The food industry has found a way to make products, sweeteners and additives from one of our country's largest crops. This is a simple way to deal with surplus and no one knows about it. What's worse is that the corn used for these additives is not even food grade corn. It is excess cattle feed, turned into your lunch, dinner and breakfast.

Educate yourself on the economics of food and you'll be shocked, outraged and ready to take control of your own health!

To find out more about the economics of foods (which will be the subject of my next book!) and where these incredible numbers came from, visit http://www.LiveAwesome.com/book.

THE BUSY PERSON'S SOLUTION #6: REALIZE THAT YOUR DRINKING WATER IS KILLING YOU AND DO SOMETHING ABOUT IT!

» ACTION » PURIFY YOUR WATER... EVEN IF YOU HAVE A WELL

Drinking water is essential for your health.
Drinking purified and filtered water is essential for your optimal health!

? What's in Your Tap Water?

If you drink tap water, stop. Get a water filter. There are poisons in your water that have been affecting you at varying levels your entire life.

! Don't listen to what people say about what's kind of safe and what's kind of not safe. Just don't drink the water.

You know how they say New York tap water is the best water in the world? BS. It has chlorine, fluoride, and numerous other metals and added chemicals that can really mess up your body.

Get a purification system now and enjoy water as it should be. I never took this seriously until I filled up a bottle of water from the tap to go running. When I was out on the trails and before I was about to take my first sip, I smelled a very strong scent of chlorine from the bottle. The smell was so strong that if someone had told me they switched my bottle with one filled with pool water I would not have second-guessed them. I bought a water filtration system and a shower filter the next day.

Chlorine causes scarring of the arteries. When the arteries scar, cholesterol now has something to attach itself to. This is what clogs arteries. So basically tap water, pools, and hot tubs help you clog your arteries.

Along with chlorine, there are hundreds of other chemicals in your tap water.

Here are just a few:

- Fluoride
- Pipe Corrosion
- Pesticides
- Oils
- Gasoline Residues
- Prescription Drugs
- Harmful Bacteria

! Contrary to what your dentist has told you... fluoride is NOT good for you.

The damaging effects of fluoride have been published since the 1960s. In America, we still put fluoride in our drinking water, while countries in Europe have completely banned the use of it.

Fluoride damages your genes and it is mind-blowing to wonder why throughout my childhood none of the dentists who gave me a fluoride cleaning knew or warned me of the nasty effects of the chemical.

What's equally amusing is that my dentist has stopped using the fluoride washes, clearly because of the knowledge he has, and yet public water companies are still putting this poison in our water!

The amount of fluoride you need to ingest to start affecting your genes does not need to be significant—as little as 0.6 parts per million of fluoride produces chromosomal damage in human white blood cells.

Many public water systems have 0.6 parts per million of fluoride or more... even in California!

What's worse is that the American Dental Association still recommends fluoride to prevent cavities! They still recommend that 0.7 to 1.2 parts per million are acceptable levels to stop cavities.

Regardless of what the ADA says, when you drink water with fluoride, you're taking in a chemical that damages your genes!

I'm not willing to sit around and take chances—nor should you.

You May Think Your Well Water is Safe...

If you have well water, you need to watch out for bacteria and other chemicals. Get your well tested and you will sleep easier knowing that everything is clear.

I was speaking to an ecologist who sells filtrations systems about a family he had dealt with. They started to get sick and no one knew what it was. I mean really sick—hospital sick. They finally tested their water and found out that the level of uranium in their well water was through the roof.

High levels of uranium cause irreparable kidney damage and failure. This stuff is lethal.

Get your water tested. Know what's there and take the proper steps to get yourself clean drinking water.

You're Being Tricked By The Bottled Water Companies

If you're drinking bottled water, read the labels. Companies will add minerals as well and try to disguise the source of the water.

There are many different companies out there that are using water from the tap that you may think is actually spring water. When you see the word "Filtered" you should be suspicious.

I'd consider avoiding the Pepsi and Coke products, Aquafina and Desani, these are taken from metropolitan water sources. Fiji, Trinity, Volvic and Evian are some that I recommend above others.

How Much Water?

You need to drink half your body weight in ounces a day. If you're 100 pounds, drink 50 ounces of water. This might vary, as ultimately it's up to you to find out for yourself.

Drinking 64 ounces a day (Eight 8-ounce glasses) for everyone doesn't cut it. It could be too much for a very small person and too little for a bigger person.

For those of you who have heard of the studies about over-hydration, also called water excess or water intoxication—please understand that these warnings are for extreme athletes who compete at marathon, ultramarathon, ironman triathlons, and other 3-7 day adventure races. When you exercise for over 2-3 hours straight then you need to start worrying about electrolyte replacement. If you drink too much water and don't replace your electrolytes then you have a problem. Your muscles lose the ability to move electrical current and your body fails. This does not mean you need to go out and buy Gatorade or worry about electrolyte pills if you are working out 30 minutes a day. Eat a banana and you'll be fine. If you are still worried, eat two bananas! Only if you are exercising for more than two to three hours straight, should you search for some electrolyte solutions that are not poisonous (have tons of sugars and chemicals in them—just about every sports drink).

» ACTIVITY » FIND OUT THE BEST FILTER FOR YOU AND GET IT TODAY!

I am not an expert in water filters. I have included reviews of systems on my website and contact information for people who know more than me.

The reason I have not listed them all here is because I want to give you the most up-to-date information. I just finished reading a book with some resources in the back. I contacted some of the names and half were no longer in business. This is the challenge of the written word!

For resources on how to get your water tested, what filters are best, and what else is in your water visit my website http://www.LiveAwesome.com/book.

THE BUSY PERSON'S SOLUTION #7: GET THE GUNK OUT OF YOUR PIPES BEFORE IT'S TOO LATE.

» ACTION » CLEANSE YOUR COLON

Chances are your body has accumulated a few environmental, food-based, or chemical toxins over the years. Getting rid of them with a cleanse is essential to optimal health.

There are many ways to cleanse. I'm not going to make it complicated. I recommend one simple cleanse to start that is quick, easy, doesn't require any appointments or require you to sit at home on the couch all day—weak and worn down.

Why a Colon/Digestive Track Cleanse?

Your colon and digestive system have been taxed with processed foods, pesticides, bacteria and hundreds of other chemicals.

To protect itself, your digestive system builds up mucous layers in your intestines, which can cause poor mineral and nutrient absorption. This, in turn, causes more hunger, nutrient deficiencies and general poor health.

 Get rid of the mucous, get your health back!

A colon cleanse will remove some or all of this mucous and let your insides function like they should.

Good news is that you can do a colon cleanse easily and in a way that is completely non-invasive—so I'm not talking about enemas and colonics.

I've heard my clients tell me that when they do a colon cleanse they are quite shocked to see what comes out. You probably will be too. They are also shocked at how clean and clear they're skin looks—it glows.

If you run into anyone who tells you that you don't need to clean your colon, ask them if they've ever seen the foul smelling, otherworldly, black colored stool—that I've seen myself and have heard others explain—that is excreted when some people do a colon cleanse.

I know for a fact that they haven't, because if they did, they'd believe in colon cleanses!

There are other types of cleanses, but for now, start with the easiest and most important. Then you can explore further afterwards.

An Important Note on Any Cleansing: If you're changing your lifestyle, cleansing, changing the foods you're eating or introducing new foods into your diet, your body might struggle at first to make sense of what is going on.

Chances are, if you've never cleansed your system there is a significant amount of junk inside and your body will want to get it out. In order to release toxins from your tissues and organs, your body will have to put them into your blood stream to transport them out.

What this means simply is that with all those poisons floating around in your blood stream, you might feel worse before you feel better.

Some common cleansing side effects are:

- Low Energy
- Headache
- Lightheadedness
- Fatigue
- Constipation
- Diarrhea
- Gas/Bloating
- Moodiness
- Anger, Sadness
- *And, eventually, feeling absolutely fantastic!*

» Activity » Start Your Internal Spring Cleaning

First, don't let all this talk about the colon and the digestive system disgust or embarrass you. Everyone has a colon, so you're no different from the next person.

The great news about this type of cleansing is that you don't have to do enemas or colonics (if you're uncomfortable with them). Good bowel cleanses can be found in pill form at the local health food store and are usually have a 5-10 day protocol that is easy to follow. If you don't use the help of the local store and decide to look for yourself, a good bowel cleanse will have ingredients like senna, cassia, cayenne, bentonite clay, psyllium husk, and aloe.

You can also go online to order Dr. Richard Schulze's 5 Day Bowel Detox that I personally recommend: www.herbdoc.com.

So don't be shy! Your colon will thank you. If you are too shy to go to the store and ask what they have, then go on the internet and take a look. I recommend a few products on my site as well.

Plus… it doesn't have to be spring to clean out your pipes! You can do it any time!

For more information on bowel cleanses and other cleanses, visit http://www.LiveAwesome.com/book.

PHENOMENAL HEALTH AND FITNESS SECRET
BODYWEIGHT EXERCISES ARE THE MOST EFFECTIVE AND EFFICIENT STRENGTH AND STRETCHING EXERCISES ON THE PLANET

One of the biggest reasons the industry doesn't want you to know that bodyweight exercises are some of the best you can do is because no one can make any money selling them—they require no equipment!

What is a bodyweight exercise? It is an exercise that builds cardiovascular and muscular strength using only your own body weight. Simple bodyweight exercises that you've heard of before are pushups and pull ups.

But these are not the only ones. In the world of bodyweight exercises there are 100's of ways to push around your own weight safely and for people of all levels of fitness.

! **Bodyweight exercises are also extremely efficient. They can stretch, strengthen and increase your stamina all at the same time. This is the ultimate solution for the busy person.**

Below you'll find seven essential bodyweight exercises that you can start doing today. You don't even need to do many before you realize how fantastic these exercises are for your heart, your health, and your strength.

THE BUSY PERSON'S SOLUTION #8: SAVE HOURS OF YOUR TIME USING THESE 7 EQUIPMENT-FREE AND SUPER-EFFICIENT EXERCISES

» ACTION » DO THESE BODY WEIGHT EXERCISES

These are the 7 staple exercises that we give our clients.

These exercises—done together—work almost every single muscle in the body.

They are easy to do, quick and efficient. I love efficient exercise. It is perfect for the busy person like you.

You can do them all at once or one a day. It doesn't matter. These seven exercises will work you out in ways you've never felt before—and since this is the case, I want to be sure you take it easy at first.

I want you to learn from my past mistakes. The goal is not to be sore after a workout. The goal is to feel fantastic!

Underneath each exercise and description are suggestions for different levels of fitness. You should start at the beginner level—no matter how strong or in shape you are—the first time, wait a day, see if you're sore and then decide if you should move to the next level.

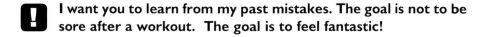

Those who do not find time for exercise will have to find time for illness.

— Earl of Derby

Exercise #1: Tai Chi Twist

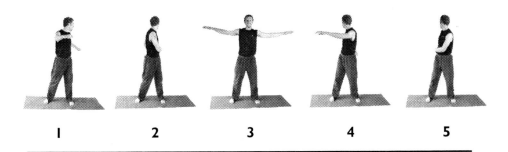

| 1 | 2 | 3 | 4 | 5 |

The Tai-Chi twist is a great exercise to loosen your spine, get your blood flowing, work on your obliques and aid in digestion.

1. Stand with slightly bent knees shoulder width apart. Place your hands at your sides and relax your limbs.
2. From here begin twisting your waist back and forth in a circular manner, and let the centrifugal force from the twisting move your arms back and forth.
3. When you pick up some speed your arms should whip around and then slap at your front and back simultaneously as you can see in the second picture.

Beginner: 2 X 30 Seconds	Intermediate: 2 X 45 Seconds	Advanced: 2 X 60 Seconds

Exercise #2: Merry-Go-Round

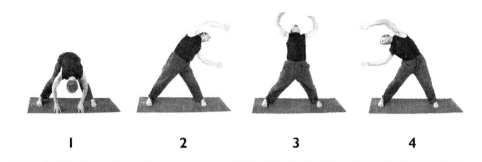

| 1 | 2 | 3 | 4 |

Merry-Go-Rounds are fantastic for your entire body. They work your hamstrings, back, arms, abs, and hip flexors. They also can get your breathing a little heavy. Don't do too many of these the first day. You'll know why soon enough!

1. Start with your legs spread and your hands in front of you touching the ground. Your knees should be barely bent.

2. Inhale as you swing your entire body to the right, keeping your hips facing straight ahead.

3. Continue your swing to the back, leaning backwards and letting your neck stay loose. At this point you will not be able to inhale anymore.

4. Exhale once you pass the middle point and move your swing to the left.

5. Come back down to the start.

6. Repeat, except start by going the other way first.
   (Each time out and back = 1 Rep)

Beginner: 2 X 10 reps	Intermediate: 3 X 10 reps	Advanced: 3 X 15 reps

Exercise #3: Easy Bridge (Beginner)

The easy bridge is a good way to work yourself into a full bridge. Once you do this for a couple of weeks you'll find your flexibility will increase and your spine will open up allowing more range of motion. For all of us, we could use a little more motion in our spines. They are not supposed to be rigid... they should be flexible and move fluidly.

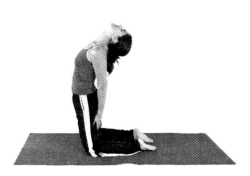

1. Start by kneeing on the ground.

2. Tilt your head back and then start curling backwards. Loosen your abs and your quadriceps for more range of motion. Try not to bend any further at the knees.

3. Use your hands on your thighs to support yourself if you need to.

4. Hold as long as you can!

5. Breathe naturally.

Beginner	Intermediate	Advanced
2 X 15 Seconds	2 X 30 Seconds	4 X 30 Seconds

Exercise #3: Half Bridge (Intermediate)

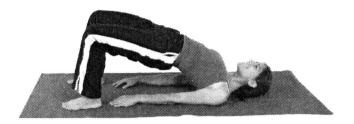

The half bridge is one step further toward the full bridge (or wheel). It flexes your spine just like the easy bridge and gets you used to being on the ground for the full bridge.

1. Start with your back on the ground and your hands at your sides. Your feet should be shoulder width apart.

2. Lift your hips up to the sky and bring your hands underneath you.

3. Bend at the back and try to bring your chest to your chin.

4. Be sure not to let your knees kick out to far. They should be straight at all times during the bridge with the same distance from each other as your feet have. If you need to, squeeze you inner thighs to make sure they are in proper position.

5. Hold as long as possible!

6. Breathe naturally.

Beginner	Intermediate	Advanced
2 X 15 Seconds	**2 X 30 Seconds**	**3 X 30 Seconds**

Exercise #3: Full Bridge (Advanced)

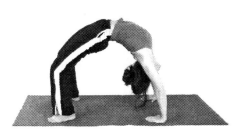

This gymnast pose is one of the best. It helps with digestion and circulation, and works your legs, abs, lower back, upper back, arms, chest, abs, and neck! The longer you can hold this pose the closer you are to maximum energy potential! Think about how quickly and unimpeded your blood with flow through your healthy and strong muscles, giving you loads of oxygen, increasing your senses and your quality of life!

This exercise will help back pain by strengthening your stabilizing muscles! You might have some difficulty even getting into the pose at first, but in a few weeks you'll be surprised at how easy it can be!

Many people cannot do this exercise right away. If you cannot, try the "Easy Bridge" or the "Half Bridge" first until you are comfortable with bending your back like this.

1. Start with your back on the ground and your hands behind your shoulders—palms facing out. Your feet should be shoulder width apart.

2. Simultaneously lift your hips and push up with your arms to form the bridge.

3. Try to look at your feet with your head!

4. Be sure not to let your knees kick out too far. They should be straight at all times during the bridge with the same distance from each other as your feet have. If you need to, squeeze you inner thighs to make sure they are in proper position.

5. Make sure you breathe naturally during this exercise.

6. Hold as long as you can! (If you can hold this pose for a minute your core is getting super strong!)

Beginner 2 X 10 Seconds	Intermediate 3 X 15 Seconds	Advanced 3 X 30 Seconds

Exercise #4: Bear Squats

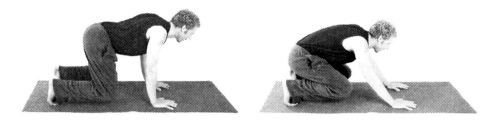

| 1 | 2 |

Bear Squats are great for your whole body! They work your legs, middle and upper body all at once and at the same time get your heart rate up!

1. Start on all fours on the ground.

2. Lift your knees about 2 inches of the ground so they are suspended.

3. Crouch back and sit on your calves (Keeping your knees 2 inches off the ground).

4. Then using your leg strength, push yourself back to the starting position. (Still keeping your knees off the ground.)

5. Repeat quickly.

6. Breathe in when you rock back, out when you spring forward.

Beginner	Intermediate	Advanced
2 Sets of 8	**3 Sets of 10**	**4 Sets of 20**

Exercise #5: Downward Dog / Upward Dog

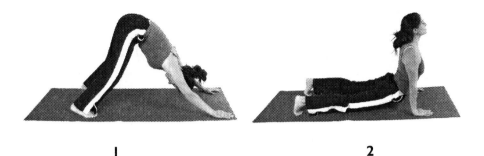

| 1 | 2 |

Downward Dog / Upward Dog is borrowed from the East. This exercise does not only work your entire upper body, it increases flexibility in the spine and increases stamina. Try these to replace regular pushups and see how quickly you will increase your upper body strength.

1. Start with your hands shoulder width apart.

2. Your feet should be on the floor at shoulder width or wider, depending on your flexibility.

3. Start with your butt in the air and your head looking back to your heels.

4. Drop your hips down to the ground, curling your back.

5. Look straight ahead and inhale.

6. Push back toward your heels again and keeping your ARMS STRAIGHT return to the start position.

Beginner	Intermediate	Advanced
2 Sets of 8	3 Sets of 10	4 Sets of 20

Exercise #6: Yoga Squats

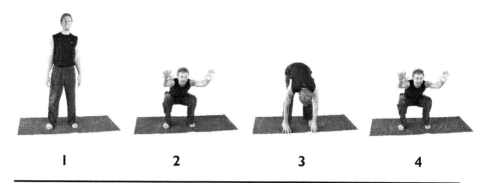

| 1 | 2 | 3 | 4 |

This squat alternative is nice on the knees and great for the heart.

1. Start with feet shoulder width apart.

2. Squat down into a catcher's stance with your hands out in front of you to balance. Breathe in.

3. Lift up your butt to the ceiling and touch your toes. Breathe out.

4. Squat back down into a catcher's stance with your hands out in front of you to balance. Breathe in.

5. Stand up and bring your hands to your side. Breathe out.

6. Repeat!

Beginner	Intermediate	Advanced
2 Sets of 8	**3 Sets of 10**	**4 Sets of 15**

Exercise #7: Rise and Shine

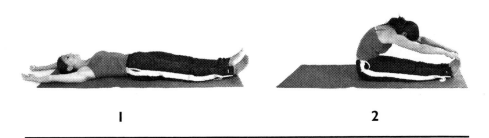

| 1 | 2 |

This form of sit-up doesn't let you cheat! You have to focus on using only your abs to lift you upright. When you get better at these, you will notice your abs becoming rock solid and your balance and posture getting better!

1. Lie on the floor with your arms at your sides.

2. Inhale as you use your abdominal muscles to pull yourself trying not to let your heels and legs come off the floor.

3. Come up and try to touch your toes.

4. Exhale as you return to start slowly making sure you don't arch your back when you return to the start position.

5. Repeat.

Beginner 2 Sets of 10	Intermediate 4 Sets of 10	Advanced 6 Sets of 10

» Activity» Start Using an EASY System to Track and Plan your Workouts

I'd like you to keep track of what you do and it doesn't have to be complicated.

Your life is complicated enough.

We've created a revolutionary and very easy to use point system to help you keep track of your activity.

The system is revolutionary for its simplicity. Too many systems figure in too many variables making them hard to follow, rigid, repetitive and boring.

The basis of our system is to get you to move—not to be concerned about how many calories you're burning.

Here's how it works.

- Make a copy of the worksheet that I have on the next page.
  (Or download it on our website: http://www.LiveAwesome.com/book)
- Do any bodyweight exercise in this book and when you do, mark 1 point on the worksheet. Each exercise you do—no matter how long, or how many reps—equals one point.
- The exercises do not have to be from this book for the system to work. If you do other exercises, mark them down as 1 point. It can be a stretch or a set of pushups. Doesn't matter.
- Walking, running, yoga and any other activities work as well. If you do any type of activity that brings your heart rate up, mark down 1 point for every five minutes of exercise. So if you walk for five minutes, mark 1 point. If you do yoga for 20 minutes mark 4 points.
- For beginners, strive to get 25-35 points a week. Intermediates, 45-55. Advanced, 65 or more.

If you want to spice it up and see a list of 100 other exercises that you can do with no or little equipment, visit http://www.LiveAwesome.com/book.

THE BUSY PERSON'S POINT TRACKER

Week	Point Goal	Mon	Tues	Wed	Thurs	Fri	Sat	Sun	Point Total
example	30	5	6	10	4	3	2	0	30
Comments:									

1 Exercise = 1 Point   5 Min of Activity (Walk, Run, Yoga, Etc.) = 1 Point

THE BUSY PERSON'S POINT TRACKER

Week	Point Goal	Mon	Tues	Wed	Thurs	Fri	Sat	Sun	Point Total
Comments:									

1 Exercise = 1 Point   5 Min of Activity (Walk, Run, Yoga, Etc.) = 1 Point

THE BUSY PERSON'S POINT TRACKER

Week	Point Goal	Mon	Tues	Wed	Thurs	Fri	Sat	Sun	Point Total
Comments:									

1 Exercise = 1 Point   5 Min of Activity (Walk, Run, Yoga, Etc.) = 1 Point

PHENOMENAL HEALTH AND FITNESS SECRET
YOU DON'T NEED TO LIFT WEIGHTS, EVER.

Weight lifting can do more harm than good.

The First Reason Weight Lifting Could be Hurting You:
The Approach

Weight lifting can be bad for you because it carries the "no pain, no gain" mentality along with it, no matter how you cut it.

If you get on a strength training program, it is inevitable that eventually you'll want to lift more weight and get bigger muscles. More and more weight means more and more stress on your skeletal and muscular systems.

I did it over and over again when I was younger. Each time I realized how much bigger I had gotten, I stopped and had to reverse the inflexibility and imbalances I created.

The Second Reason Weight Lifting Could be Hurting You:
It Causes Imbalance

Most weight lifting focuses on isolating certain muscles—this is a direct cause of imbalance.

If you pile a bunch of rocks on a 2X4 that's spanned across two saw horses, the thing's going to bend—or possibly break. This is the same principle with your body. If you over load one group of muscles, then another will suffer greatly.

I'm sure you've seen a program that tells you to start at a weight that is comfortable for you then increase gradually.

How do you know that the weight you're starting with is good for you? How do you know when to increase?

If you increase the weight you're using when one muscle group is stronger than another, then the other muscle group will lag behind. If you really push when you're lifting your chest muscles and slack off on your back, you're putting strain on your body and creating major imbalances.

These imbalances lead to pain and discomfort down the road that can be avoided by doing bodyweight exercises that work muscles complementary to others and only require your own weight.

The Third Reason Weight Lifting Could be Hurting You:
Anaerobic/Adrenal Stress

Weight lifting creates stress on your body.

When you lift weights, you are using your anaerobic energy system which uses sugar as a fuel. Because your body only carries 2500-3000 calories of readily available glucose in the blood stream, anaerobic activity uses these stores. The reason this sugar is stored is for emergencies (life or death situations), which is a remnant of our prehistoric past—most of us don't have to worry about running from tigers anymore. Any workout that requires 3-4 sets of 10-12 or less with moderate to heavy weight is anaerobic activity. This taxes your system, because your body and metabolic systems think they are being threatened.

This stress causes fatigue, irritability, low blood sugar, and sugar cravings, because your body is telling you that it needs to replenish its glucose stores. Glucose is your primary brain food, so you can see how important this is. Without glucose, your mind doesn't function efficiently.

What's worse about this anaerobic stress is that most of our adrenals are already taxed by every day stresses. This leads to double the stress on our body which is just downright unhealthy.

When I lifted weights, afterward I not only felt weak, but I craved sugar—a signal that my adrenals were on overload and needed more fuel. I used to think that this was how I was supposed to feel after a good workout. Maybe you feel this way too, but it's just not the case.

 At the end of a workout you should feel energized and ready to take on the world—not tired, sleepy and, craving for anything in the fridge.

THE BUSY PERSON'S SOLUTION #9: STOP TAKING THE SUPERMARKET MULTIVITAMIN AND START SUPPLEMENTING WITH WHOLE FOODS

» ACTION » SUPPLEMENT YOUR DIET WITH WHOLE FOODS, SUPERFOODS AND WHOLE FOOD MINERAL PRODUCTS

Multivitamins are formulated on averages. You are not an average.

Most big brand multivitamins are synthetically made, and many times they don't resemble anything your body makes or needs naturally. Worse, they are eliminated just as quickly as they are put into the body. (So yes, your bright, lemon-lime Gatorade colored urine is your $10 a bottle multi going down the drain).

These big vitamin companies are taking the "mayonnaise approach"— a term courtesy of my chiropractor—which means that in one sweeping motion they've produced a vitamin product and made you believe that it covers all the bases.

Unfortunately for this type of science, you're not like the next person. You eat different things, your metabolism is different and you have different activity levels.

The multivitamin cannot be sufficient for the runner AND the couch potato. It's impossible.

So here's the challenge—since the JAMA reversed it's stance on whole food nutrition in 2002, stating that we must supplement because our conventional foods are deficient in nutrients—what do we do to get the minerals we need?

You can do all or a combination of these four things…

Eat Whole Organic Foods

Organics generally have more nutrients than conventional foods and are grown in more nutrient rich soils. When soils are showered with synthetic fertilizers the plant will grow, but will not grow with an optimal amount of minerals. The natural minerals found in the soils will eventually become more and more diluted because each time a new crop is planted the crop uses those trace minerals.

If you haven't made the switch to organics yet, you should consider starting right away.

Eat Superfoods

Most of the superfoods I listed in the superfoods section are highly mineralized foods and will help replace the nutrient deficiencies you may have. Add them to your diet and then see how you feel. If your mood increases and your energy levels soar, you're on the right track.

Juice Vegetables and Fruits

Juicing vegetables will concentrate minerals and enzymes into a fantastic tasting drink. The more you juice the better you look, which makes this a very important and effective way to get the minerals you need in your diet.

Use a Whole Food Supplement

A whole food supplement is a supplement made directly from whole foods. These are made from whole fruits, vegetables, herbs, roots and other plants that contain a wide range of vitamins and minerals. The difference between a whole food supplement and a multivitamin supplement is that the whole food supplement is made from real foods in their natural form. The nutrients are not synthetic or derived from a whole food source. The source is the actual food.

The reason these are fantastic products is because your body recognizes them for what they are... real food!

Some great whole food supplements are:
- Dr. Schulze's "Superfood"
- Mitchell May's "Pure Synergy"
- Jameth Sheridan's "Nature's First Food"

(You can find each one of them by an online web search or you check my website for more info.)

 For the Scientific... Get Tested

If you're still the extremely scientific type, then get tested by a nutritionist or doctor to see the deficiencies that you have. Just remember that the recommended, acceptable, and optimal levels of vitamins and nutrients for these tests are based on scientific studies that may or may not have used unreliable sample groups to represent the population as a whole.

Again, as I've mentioned before, do your own research and give it a shot!

» ACTIVITY » START SUPPLEMENTING WITH WHOLE FOODS AND PRODUCTS TODAY!

I can't give you specific nutritional advice for your specific needs. That's not what I do. What I can do is give you information on how to find out for yourself.

Here are some steps you can take:

1. Pick one of these five whole food supplementation recommendations you think might fit into your schedule.
2. Consult a nutritionist or doctor if you have questions.
3. Take action.

When you take action, you will get feedback from your body which will tell you if the product is working or not. If it works, then make it a part of your everyday experience. If it doesn't, move on to the next recommendation.

I've given some examples here for you to try. To see the extensive section of nutritional and whole food supplements that doctors and nutritionists recommend and have the highest standards of quality, visit http://www.LiveAwesome.com/book.

Note: The reason most products are posted on my site and not in this book, is because products and companies change, I hesitate to put that information here in the book because I don't want it to be outdated. I want to keep a hawk's eye on these products and make sure you're getting the best information out there!

THE BUSY PERSON'S SOLUTION #10: DRINK YOUR VEGGIES FOR A QUICK MEAL AND MAXIMUM HEALTH

» ACTION » BUY A JUICE TODAY!

I've heard different advice as what is the best thing to do right now to change your diet. Eat less carbs, eat less fat, eat less...

This is all great advice, but there is one single piece of advice that transcends all of these tips--and that is to have one fresh vegetable juice a day.

! **There is no better way to get whole nutrients, get more energy and feel fantastic than to drink at least one vegetable juice a day.**

Good news for the busy person is that you will find juicers at most local health food stores, so you'll never have to clean the machine and prepare them yourself!

When you juice a vegetable you separate the enzymes, vitamins and minerals from the fiber. This gives you a concentrated mix that will put you bounds ahead in your health and fitness.

Juicing can be better than other types of supplementation because the nutrients are still fresh and none of them are damaged from heat, cold (refrigeration and freezing), exposure or any other factor that can deplete their potency.

The effects of adding fresh fruit and vegetable juices to your diet can be seen in days. Many people I have worked with tell me their skin and blemishes clear up, scratches and injuries heal faster, and overall energy levels rise dramatically.

If you've never had a fresh vegetable juice—and I don't mean the bottled juices that you see in the grocery stores—I want you to go to the local health store and see if they make them. Most of them do have juicers on the premises. Ask for something simple and try it. You'll be amazed at how good it tastes!

If you've already juiced before either wipe the dust of your old machine or go out and buy a new one. A juicer can run anywhere from $80.00-$4000.00, but to start don't spend a bunch of money. A centrifugal juicer is fine. This type of juicer will liquefy any hard vegetable and some leafy vegetables as well. There are other types—press, screw and wheatgrass—but this is the best way to start.

Start with pleasant tasting vegetables and fruits. Carrots, apples, celery, cucumbers, tomatoes and grapes are the best for beginners. Mix them together or just have them alone. Once you start to enjoy fresh juice then you can explore other combinations and vegetables. If you're anything like me, you probably experiment a bit with different flavors and ingredients not knowing what to expect!

If you are struggling to find different ingredients… beets, kale, spinach or cabbage are just a few to try in your next mixture.

Try putting garlic in your juice to boost your immune system, ginger to aid in digestion or cilantro to give it an added fresh flavor for the summer!
Be sure to buy produce that is organically grown. These fruits and vegetables are loaded with more nutrients and have none of the pesticides you'll find in non-organic foods.

Also be sure to clean your juicer after each use to avoid any mold growth that will compromise all the wonderful benefits of fresh juices.

» ACTIVITY » GO AHEAD, TRY IT!

Here are some recipes that any novice will enjoy and any health food store will have!

1. Just Carrot
2. Just Apple
3. Carrot, Apple and Celery
4. Cucumber, Celery, Carrot
5. Parsley, Beet, Celery, Apple and Ginger
6. Kale, Carrot, Apple and Parsley

These are pretty mild juices. If you're making them yourself, the more carrot and apple you add the sweeter and more palatable they will be!

Good luck and enjoy!

...Oh! If you're at a juice bar, try a shot of wheatgrass as well!

For more recipes, juicers that will work for you and other juicing related sources, visit http://www.LiveAwesome.com/book.

PHENOMENAL HEALTH AND FITNESS SECRET
DON'T LISTEN TO THE FAT GUY TELL YOU WHAT TO EAT, HOW TO EXERCISE AND HOW TO STAY HEALTHY—YOU KNOW EXACTLY WHAT'S RIGHT FOR YOU

Don't listen to the fat guy's advice.

I say this with all seriousness. If you want to be in fantastic health, search for your mentors, find the healthiest people out there and ask them what they do. They will give you good answers.

You might not like the answers they give, but they most likely are the solutions that will get you the results you need.

Don't listen to the health advice that Jim, Sally or your parents or your friends give you, unless they are a fantastic picture of health. You wouldn't trust your finances to an impoverished accountant, why would you do any less for your body?

I've seen a bunch of overweight nutritionists and trainers in my time. This is a sure sign they're not the best people to listen to. This doesn't mean their information is wrong, it just means that they might give you advice that will send you further off track. Stay away!

What's even more deceptive to this secret is that I've seen a ton of muscle-bound men and women who suffer from excruciating back pain everyday. You'd never know it—because they look fantastic—but they hurt all the time. You don't want to look like them, and then realize—firsthand—how they feel on a day-to-day basis.

Pick your mentors carefully. Don't just take anyone's advice. If a family member tells you something is good for you, ask them why and how they heard about it. They'll probably say from someone at work or on the news. Don't believe it unless it's coming from the horse's mouth.

Your life is too short to be listening to health and fitness advice from people who aren't in great mental and physical shape.

This doesn't mean that you should look down on your friends and family for being misinformed, it means get out there, find the information that is going to help you and then educate THEM!

THE BUSY PERSON'S SOLUTION #11: USE YOUR HEART AS YOUR GUIDE AND SAVE A BOATLOAD OF TIME

» ACTION » FIGURE OUT YOUR FAT BURNING HEART RATE

Now that you're already moving, I'm going to let you in on a little fat burning secret.

 Keeping your heart rate at a certain level for an extended period of time is truly the one scientific fact that no-fail will burn calories.

When your metabolism is sped up, you're burning sugar as fuel. And when you use the Fat Burning Heart Rate system, you'll be burning fat.

Note: You do not have to use this system at all. If you find that it is too much, too confusing, or just don't want to be bothered, you can skip this section and still get results. The FBHR system is to help you be more efficient with your workouts, because I know how busy you are!

Why a Fat Burning Heart Rate?

I'm going to spare you the scientifics. Your body has three different fuel systems. The one we're focusing on is the aerobic system. This system uses fatty acids, glycerol and oxygen for fuel. Fatty acids and glycerol are formed when your body fat tissue (adipose) is broken down.

Your body tunes into this particular system when you're operating at a steady and elevated heart rate, which I call your Fat Burning Heart Rate.

If you exercise at too high a heart rate, you then will use the anaerobic system, which burns glucose and creates lactic acid. This is the feeling you get when your muscles burn. This creates stress on the body and also creates sugar cravings, because after you are done exercising, your body needs to replenish your sugar energy stores.

So for our purposes, fat burning is where it's at.

Exercises That Will Get You Burning Fat (But Not Limited To):

- Running
- Walking
- Kayaking
- Hiking
- Biking
- Spinning (Stay in your FBHR!)
- Rowing
- Yoga (Stay in your FBHR.)
- Pilates
- Aerobic Dance
- Martial Arts
- Wood Chopping
- Moderate/High Intensity Yard Work
  (Lawn moving, raking leaves, lifting and hauling)

 Motivation is what gets you started. Habit is what keeps you going.
— *Jim Ryun*

» ACTIVITY » LEARN HOW TO USE YOUR FAT BURNING HEART RATE FOR MAXIMUM EFFICIENCY

All you need is a digital watch (or one with a second hand) and two fingers.

Step One: Make sure you've been sitting for at least 60 minutes or so.

Step Two: Place your index and middle fingers of your right hand on the soft left side of your opposite wrist—below the thumb. You should feel a pulse.

Step Three: Count the number of beats over a 60 second time period.

Step Four: That is your Resting Heart Rate (RHR). Write that number below.

Your Resting Heart Rate (RHR) is: _____

Note: Generally RHR is in the 50-80 range. 70-80 Beats per minute is on the high side, so if you get a reading like this, wait 15 minutes or so and try again. If it is still that high, you might consider going to the doctor for a check up. Elevated blood pressure could be a sign of a more serious medical condition.

How to Figure Your Fat Burning Heart Rate (FBHR)

Don't worry, there's only a little bit of math! Just plug the numbers into the equation and you'll get your FBHR!

220 – [Your Age] – [Your RHR] = _____
Take the answer from above and use it in the next equation:

[Answer from Above] X 0.6 = _____
Again, take the answer from above and use it in the final equation:

[Answer from Above] + [Your RHR] = _____
This answer is your Fat Burning Heart Rate (FBHR)

My FBHR is: _____

Note: Your FBHR—depending on your age—should be in the 110-150 range. If it is outside of that range, check the math again to see if you made a mistake.

How to Monitor Your FBHR

You will monitor your FBHR with the same technique you used to determine your Resting Heart Rate with a few exceptions:

You still need a digital watch or one with a second hand and two fingers.

Step One: While you're exercising, stop, then immediately place your index and middle fingers of your right hand on the soft left side of your opposite wrist—below the thumb. You should feel a pulse.

Step Two: Count the number of beats over a 15 second time period.

Step Three: Multiply that number by 4.

Step Four: Start exercising again.

If your heart rate is too low, then raise the intensity, if your heart rate is too high, then slow down a bit.

You should do this routine about every 10 minutes to make sure you're on track.

Using a Heart Rate Monitor

If you want to get one, use it. If you don't, then use the quick technique and guidelines I provided above and you'll still succeed.

Again, this program is supposed to make this as easy as possible for you. If strapping on a heart rate monitor is easy, then by all means get one.

Note: Use your senses when you're exercising. If you feel dizzy, lightheaded, faint, nauseous or are experiencing pain, see a doctor. If you are unsure about how to take your pulse any nurse or doctor can show you how.

THE BUSY PERSON'S SOLUTION #12: USE THE FORCE, LUKE

» ACTION » START EXPLORING ON YOUR OWN!

I know that if you've made it this far, you're committed to your health and fitness. You've been a great student. Now it's up to you to "use the Force, Luke."

That means use what you've learned and go out on your own.

But first, I want you to take a moment, give yourself a pat on the back and take a deep breath. Relax and enjoy it. You've accomplished a lot in a very short period of time.

Now let me tell you about the next step...

It's your turn. It's up to you to be an evangelist for your own health and the health of the others around you. You know how to get started, so go out and tell everyone else how to feel as fantastic as you feel now.

Let me tell you about my goals and maybe you can join me on my ultimate quest.

I want to reach one million people with this message—maybe more. I want to show people how easy it is to exercise. I want to stop the confusion—caused by the magazines, the biased studies and the marketers—that is getting in the way of you reaching your ultimate health and fitness goals.

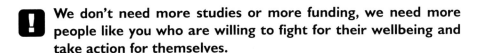 **We don't need more studies or more funding, we need more people like you who are willing to fight for their wellbeing and take action for themselves.**

Tell everyone you know about this book. Give them as gifts. If you want a bunch of them, visit the website and call us directly and we'll give you a killer deal. I want to get this book in the hands of those one million people—and more—who desperately need this advice.

Tell everyone about the website as well. It will constantly grow as the number of people who are using it as a resource grows.

This is my mission and I'd love for you to help. Maybe it can become your mission as well.

Regardless, I want to personally thank you for the time you've taken out of your busy schedule and I look forward to hearing about your success.

It's really so simple...
Take action. Get results.

Phenomenal Health and Fitness Secret
Great Health and Fitness is the Key to Fantastic Success in Whatever You Do

If you're healthy, you will succeed.

If you get out of bed everyday with a great attitude and act on your goals, you will succeed in anything that you do.

Many of our great leaders know the power of having a fit body. They might not be in the same shape as the people on the covers of the magazines (but remember what I said about them), but they know that if they move and exercise they have a better outlook and get more accomplished.

There are other reasons healthy people are successful.

- They have made a habit of activity. They take action on their goals.
- They radiate color and confidence when they walk in a room.
- They smile more.
- They don't let their food control them.
- They realize how a healthy mind affects their mind chemistry.
- They use exercise as an effective mode of stress relief.

Want to be able to do and have all those things?

Start moving today and you'll be there in no time!

WHAT? YOU HAVE QUESTIONS?!?
HERE ARE JUST A FEW FREQUENTLY ASKED QUESTIONS...

Why do you say not to listen to scientific studies? Doesn't science have its place?

Yes, science has a place. It tells us that we shouldn't eat poisons, that we need to eat different nutrients and we can test what nutrients we're deficient in or what ones we're not. Metabolic science can tell us how our bodies operate.

The scientific studies of exercise and of foods (what I've referenced as the "flavor-of-the-month" science) is slippery and with my experience and observation, it isn't helping us make good decisions. It is confusing people and paralyzing people them from getting out and moving. Even worse it is extremely daunting for a busy person to sift through.

So for now, don't use these studies that you read about in the media and journals as "absolute." Find your own truths by experimenting a little at a time and doing your own research.

I exercise everyday and I weight lift. Does this mean I should stop?

No. Keep doing what you're doing. I don't want you to stop lifting if you like it. I just want you to be aware of how lifting can affect your body. Lift consciously and take note of how you feel afterward. If you don't sense anything negative and your body recovers quickly, you don't feel inflexible or you don't have any pain afterwards, then your body can handle the type of weight lifting that you're doing.

If, on the contrary, you start feeling some of those things I mentioned before, replace a workout with a yoga class or try some cardiovascular exercise to stay in peak shape.

If you still want to lift weights, adjust how you're doing it. Change up the reps and the weight and you might find it works better for your body.

Is organic really that much better for you?

Yes. (See the FDA pesticide list on my site!)

Why do you have some resources listed on your website and not in the book... do I have to pay to get on the website?

No, you don't have to pay to get on the website at all.

There are two reasons why I have you go to the website.

One is because this book is for busy people. It was originally over 400 pages, but I made a decision that busy people don't want to read a 400 page book. So I took all the essential info and put it in the book. Then I decided if you wanted to explore more about a certain topic, you could look on the site and get more info.

Secondly, I want to be able to give you the best and most up-to-date information. If I put all the information in this book and you read it in two years, things will be outdated, companies will have gone under and my recommendations may change. So to stop this from happening, I put a bunch of information on the website so I could have complete control over the information you are getting and I can be assured that it is the best possible!

Does following this system really work?

Absolutely.

What experience do you have helping people find their optimal health?

Annmarie and I—at the time of this writing—have over 10 years combined experience in athletics, exercise and results. We teach classes, speak and work one-on-one with many people of all body types and abilities.

We have committed ourselves as full-time coaches and trainers, so our ability to learn, research and challenge has given us a unique and fresh outlook on fitness and health.

We have certifications and degrees and all that other jazz, but I don't focus on that and I don't think you should either. A College, Masters, or PhD degree doesn't guarantee that anyone can give you the information that you need.

A success to me is if someone I teach succeeds—plain and simple—and people we teach (and listen!) do succeed.

Is your guarantee really 200%?

I want you to succeed. People who use this system feel better, have more energy and lose weight. So I know that if you follow the steps you will do the same.

I want to take all the risk off of you. I know how much you've spent on different programs before and I bet you wish you had that money back— I know it's happened to me. So in order to gain your trust, I offer a 200% guarantee. This program will work for you, so smile and start taking action!

I can't find my pulse to measure my heart rate.

It's in there! I promise.

Place your right pointer and middle finger on the fat part of the base of your left thumb. Drag them down the left side of your arm past your wrist and they should sink into your arm about 1-2 inches below your thumb. Feel around. You'll feel a thump! That's it!

How long should an exercise session be?

Your exercise session should be as long as the time you have to exercise! The more you move the better you feel.

This system is liberating because it does not require you to do an hour every day or a certain routine. It fits with your busy schedule and allows you the freedom to exercise when you can and know you're doing it right.

If you "Fall off" for a few weeks can you just start up again?

Yes! Of course you can. You're human. Each motion forward will give you feedback as to if it is the right motion or not. Once you realize what has happened, then you can correct yourself to get back on the right track! Let's just hope it happens sooner than later!

I exercise at a heart rate that is much higher than my (Fat Burning Heart Rate) FBHR and I haven't lost any weight. I don't feel like I'm getting a workout when I'm in my FBHR. Why am I still struggling to reach my goals?

If you take the equation for FBHR and instead of multiplying by 0.6, you multiply by 0.8, you'll find your Sugar Burning Heart Rate. This is a higher heart rate and is used to tell when you are exercising in a sugar burning mode.

When you're in this mode, your body will burn your sugar stores instead of fat and you'll have to replenish those stores after your workout. This means that you'll crave sugar and carbohydrates. Have you ever seen the tables of food after a 5K race? Doughnuts, pizza, cookies, etc. This is not good practice for fat loss.

The best advice I can give is keep your heart rate lower and trust that you're getting a workout. You'll find that your sugar and carbohydrate cravings will decrease if you workout and maintain your FBHR.

I have shoulder and neck problems, what's the best exercise routine or particular exercises for me?

The best advice I can give to you is to be mindful of your posture. Your ears should be in line with your shoulders and your shoulders should be relaxed and in line with your hips. You should not puff your chest out!

It is hard to tell you what to do exactly if I'm not there to assess the issue. But many of these problems are related to tight chest muscles and weak upper back muscles. So to start off, I would avoid any exercise that will be working your chest and also anything that requires you to lift above your head. You want to focus on stretching out that area by stretching your arms across a doorway and leaning into the room.

If the pain still persists after these suggestions, then I would check with a chiropractor or orthopedic doctor to get their opinion.

I always seem to lose weight quickly the first few weeks then it slows down—sometimes completely—why is that?

In the first few weeks of your program, your body will go through some neurological changes. These account for the increased weight loss in the beginning.

Once these changes take place, you should expect 1-2 pounds of weight loss a week, as long as you're regulating your nutritional intake!

If I start slowly and only work out 3 days a week how is that going to help me lose weight?

Good question.

When you start off slowly, you lessen the chance of injury and give your body a chance to make the neurological changes that occur when you start an exercise program.

Most importantly, we want you to make this a habit. If you go out too fast with weight loss the only goal, then your chances of gaining the weight back later on are higher. This program is geared to get you started on a life-long path of great health—it is not a quick fix program.

Keep at the program and we guarantee that you'll lose the weight and feel fantastic before you know it!

Do I need to lift weights to stop osteoporosis?

No. You can, but there are better options.

You need to do three things:

1. Cut back your sugar intake. Sugars create acidity in the body which breaks down tissues. If you put a piece of meat in acid, the acid eats away at

it. Same thing happens in your body. Acidic pH = disintegration.

2. Do strength and stretching exercises like the bodyweight exercises that I have in this book.

3. Eat superfoods that have calcium and magnesium. Cacao, pumpkin seeds and sea vegetables.

Doing all these three things will greatly improve your chances of living with healthier bones!

I'm busy! What do I eat at restaurants?

Here are a few guidelines that we use.

1. Salads. Get a salad with olive oil and lemon dressing. Ask for the oil on the side and have them bring you a couple slices of lemon. Don't eat the dressings they have at the restaurant. They have tons of sugar in them.

2. Ask for sauce on the side. If you're getting anything with sauce like Chinese or Thai see if they can put the sauce on the side for you. Then you can regulate how many calories you eat.

3. Don't order the pasta dish. They give you way too much and you're going to keep eating it!

4. Split the meal in half and then take the rest home for the next day.

5. Don't order fried foods. The oil they fry foods at restaurants—in most cases—have labels on them that say "for frying use only". I know because I used to work at a store that shared a dumpster with a restaurant. Why can't we put this oil on our salads? I don't want to know the answer!

6. Don't order sodas or juices. The amount of calories you're going to be getting is already a bunch. Don't add to it by getting drinks.

7. If you're going to eat out and you know you're going to be decadent, don't eat at McDonald's. Go to the nicest steakhouse or restaurant in town order the best meal you can possibly imagine and enjoy every single bite of it.

Chances are you'll feel better about this, than you will if you get a Big Mac and feel guilty afterwards.

Don't waste your time with fast food.

How do I exercise when I travel?

Use the same principles in this book. Just move when you can. Here are some options…

- Use the exercises in this book when you're in the hotel room.
- Use the facility if they have one.
- Take walks (Too cold? Walk in the hotel halls).
- Don't rent a car and stay within walking distance of where you need

to go.
- Use the pool.
- Stretch on the plane.
- Stop and take quick 5 minute refreshing walks at rest stops.
- There are hundreds of things! Just move!

How much stretching should I do?

I stretch when I do my bodyweight exercises and yoga. These practices both strengthen and stretch at the same time. This is extremely efficient.

I recommend to just find a little time during the day to stretch. Even if you do just one stretch, you're moving forward. A cat stretches all the time, so think about how you can do little stretches here and there throughout your day.

I think stretching in the evening is better than in the morning because your muscles are looser. This works for me. I also do not stretch before or after I run. I stretch in the evenings. This may or may not work for you, but you know what to do… try it and see!

For many more answers, travel workout routines, stretching routines and to ask your own questions, visit http://www.LiveAwesome.com/book.

APPENDIX #1: DON'T GET OVERWHELMED!!!

That was a ton of information.

If you're overwhelmed, what I want you to do now is take a deep breath. Relax.

You can start getting your health in line by doing SOMETHING. Doesn't matter what it is and you don't have to do it all at once. It has taken me a long time to eat as healthy as I do now. I don't expect you to do it in a few hours. It has taken me longer to be in the shape I'm in.

Go back into the book, flip through the pages and pick just one thing to do.

Do something small first—you don't need to go crazy! Being over-whelmed will only freeze you and scare you into inaction.

So again, if you didn't already, take a deep breath and relax. You'll be healthy in no time!

APPENDIX #2: SHARE YOUR SUCCESS STORY WITH US!

We want to know how you're doing! We do this because we want you to succeed!

So, the minute you start seeing some results, send us an email and we'll give you a special gift!

You can reach us at our website http://www.LiveAwesome.com/book.

We look forward to helping you reach your incredible fitness goals!

Kevin and Annmarie

THE BUSY PERSON'S FITNESS SOLUTION MAIL ORDER FORM

You can order direct from our website, but if you want to mail this order form and get a copy for a friend or your boss or anyone you feel is too busy to get out there and take control of their own health... then that's cool too!

Name: _____

Address: _____

City: _____ State: _____ Zip: _____

Email: _____

Book Ordering Information

Quantity: _____

Total Price: _____ ($19.95 Each + $5.50 shipping and handling)

Additional Information (Shipping, Comments, etc.):

Type of Credit Card: _____

Name on Card: _____

Credit Card Number: _____

Expiration Date: _____ / _____

Make Checks Payable to **KMG Associates, LLC**
Please allow 1-2 weeks for receipt and delivery.

Mail this form to: A Better Life Press, P.O. Box 228, Bethel, CT 06801

For wholesale pricing please visit http://www.LiveAwesome.com/book and contact us directly.

LiveAwesome.com is the Busy Person's ULTIMATE, No BS Resource for Optimal Health, Nutrition, Wellbeing and Fitness Information!

Visit www.LiveAwesome.com/book and explore Kevin Gianni and Annmarie Colameo's ultimate resource for health, fitness, and beyond. On the site, you'll find the newest and freshest information you need to *reach your optimal health in the least amount of time!*

Here are just some of the free resources you'll find:

- Over 100 exercises you can do in a space the size of your bathroom.
- Free reports and downloads that give you the information you want right away.
- MP3s and Videos for you to download.
- Our archive of informative and motivating health, fitness, and success articles.
- Great stress relief tips that will make you as cool as a cucumber in minutes.
- And all the other resources we couldn't possibly include in this book!

You can also join the "Busy Person's Optimal Health Club" which gives you exclusive access to interviews, teleseminars, our health and fitness discussion board, our monthly newsletter and—of course—Annmarie and me!

Visit http://www.LiveAwesome.com/book to find out more!